DATE DUE		

L-91

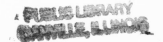

The Gift of Health

BY THE AUTHOR

The Complete Book of Sports Medicine

Total Body Training

THE GIFT OF HEALTH

WHEN FAITH AND MEDICINE AGREE — AND WHEN THEY DON'T

Richard H. Dominguez, M.D.

LIFEJOURNEY
BOOKS

DAVID C. COOK PUBLISHING CO.
ELGIN, ILLINOIS • WESTON, ONTARIO

LifeJourney Books is an imprint of David C. Cook Publishing Co.

David C. Cook Publishing Co., Elgin, Illinois 60120
David C. Cook Publishing Co. Weston, Ontario

THE GIFT OF HEALTH
© 1987 by Dr. Richard H. Dominguez

Edited by LoraBeth Norton

Cover by Edward Letwenko
Pages composed with Ready Set Go!™

First Printing, 1987
Printed in the United States of America
92 91 90 89 88 87 5 4 3 2 1

Library of Congress Cataloging in Publication Data

Dominguez, Richard H.
   The gift of health / Richard Dominguez.
    192 pages
   "LifeJourney"
   ISBN 1-555-13311-8
   1. Health—Religious aspects—Christianity. 2. Spiritual healing.
   I. Title.
BT732.D65 1987   87-20307
248'.4—dc19   CIP

— Dedication —

This book is dedicated to the mothers of my life —

• Judy — My wife. I love her dearly. She has redefined motherhood to me. She knows and loves her children and treats them as individuals. They are independent and won't ever have red underwear.

• Louise — My mother. She spoiled me. I love her more than I can ever tell her.

• Clara Musselman Macorkel — My maternal grand-mother and my spiritual mentor. I miss this gracious, lovely lady.

• Loraine Wickware — The best mother-in-law anyone could have. Now she is trapped in a body and can't communicate. My heart pains for her and her daughter.

• Salmone Valverde Dominguez — My paternal grandmother, an elegant native American. I am disappointed that I never could speak her language and get close to her.

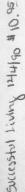

— Contents —

— Acknowledgments —

I have had the help of some good friends in this project.

- Joanne Hampe continues to encourage me to write. Her help with the manuscript has been invaluable.

- Ron Scott gave me the time in Sunday School. I never would have put it all together without that impetus.

- And my Houghton College Connection —
  Paul Mouw ('65) Any success this book has is due to his genius.
  LoraBeth (Stockin) Norton ('77) She turned my ramblings into writing and makes it read as if I were a writer.

—1—

What's a Christian to Do?

The time: the early 70s. The place: a western suburb of Chicago. Barbara and Jan, two lovely Christian girls, graduated from high school and went off to different colleges.

During her freshman year, Barbara became ill. The diagnosis wasn't clear, but it was obvious that Barbara had a progressive neurological disorder that was going to cripple her and eventually lead to her death.

Barbara attended my mother's fundamental, evangelical church. Its people prayed for Barbara over a long period of time, yet she continued to weaken. When Barbara was hospitalized, my mother would mention it to me. "Stop by and say hi to my friend Barbara." So I would make a social call to see this young girl, who was at times on oxygen and on a respirator.

Jan, her high school friend, went on to finish college. Eventually she married and became a lab technician in a Minnesota hospital, a prestigious medical center carrying on extensive cancer research.

Meanwhile, Barbara's condition grew worse. Her bladder and bowel function became paralyzed, so that she required a catheter to drain her bladder and an osteomy to drain her bowels. She became wheelchair

bound, bedridden, and finally began slipping in and out
of a coma. Clearly, Barbara did not have long to live
Much prayer continued to go up on her behalf.

During several hospitalizations, Barbara was placed
in a "no code" category—meaning that if she stopped
breathing, she would be permitted to die "naturally"
rather than having her life revived and maintained by
artificial means. Several times it seemed that death was
days, if not hours, away, but Barbara somehow survived.
She remained bedridden, dependent on all kinds of
medical equipment.

During one of Barbara's better spells, I was formally
consulted to evaluate progressive ankle and foot deformities caused by the paralysis in her lower extremities.
Though it had been months since she had walked, her
parents and her physician wanted to know if there was
anything I could do to correct these foot deformities.

When I examined her, she had marked atrophy and
weakness in her lower extremities. Her legs were almost completely paralyzed. Her feet and ankles were assuming a grotesque position that would make walking
difficult and soon impossible, even if she had the
strength to permit it in the first place. The deformities
could be corrected with at least one major operation on
each extremity, requiring three months of casting on
each leg.

I had a long conversation with Barbara. She lay in
bed, breathing through an oxygen tube; I sat on a chair
beside the bed. I told her that while technically I could
correct her feet and ankles, I personally didn't feel it
would be worth it to her. It had been months since she
had walked, and her disease was clearly progressive; the
hope of walking did not appear to be realistic. To under-
go two major reconstructive operations over a six-

month period of time, when she was never going to walk again anyway, didn't seem very sensible. Why should she subject herself to the pain and discomfort—and risks—of that surgery? (I didn't even mention the challenge of finding a willing anesthesiologist for elective major orthopedic surgery on someone who could not even breathe comfortably without the aid of oxygen equipment.) Barbara agreed with my analysis, saying that she and her parents just wanted to hear what her options were.

Jan's Plight

Meanwhile, back in Minnesota, Jan began to feel sick. When she didn't feel good for a longer period of time than she thought was normal for a "cold," she began to wonder if she had mononucleosis. As a laboratory technician, it was easy to run blood tests on herself without even consulting her physician. With the aid of some friends, Jan examined her own blood cells. To their horror, they immediately recognized the presence of grossly abnormal cells—leukemic cells—in Jan's blood.

Jan's mother, Evon, worked with me as an operating room nurse. A devout evangelical Christian, Evon kept me informed about Jan's illness and asked for prayer. Jan's church in Minnesota and her mother's in Illinois united in their appeals to the Lord for Jan's healing.

In addition, Jan had access to some of the world's greatest authorities on leukemia. She underwent vigorous, intensive chemotherapy, but she had an especially virulent form of the disease and did not respond to chemotherapy. She was advised to have a bone marrow transplant. After much thought and prayer, she underwent the painful treatment.

Sometimes, when Jan's mother and I were alone in

the hospital coffee lounge, we wondered aloud why two lovely young women, in the prime of their lives, were struck down by severe, apparently fatal illnesses. Neither of us had an explanation that satisfied us. We couldn't see any good that could come from either Jan's or Barbara's illnesses.

At first Jan's bone marrow transplant appeared to be working. She had been so weakened by the chemotherapy preceding it that she had been unable to return to work. When her weakness lasted longer that it "should have," she asked her friends to do another blood test. The cancerous leukemic cells were back.

After long talks with her husband, with the hematologist with whom she worked, and with the Lord through prayer, Jan announced that she would not have any further chemotherapy. The couple realized death was inevitable, and Jan was tired of being sick from the treatments. In a heartbreaking conversation with her mother, Jan said that she accepted this as the Lord's will, although she did not understand it, and she was at peace.

Without chemotherapy to stem the tide, Jan deteriorated rapidly. Back in Illinois, Evon's heart was breaking. There was nothing I could do or say to relieve the pain.

One Sunday Night

At the same time, Barbara came back into the hospital. This time, it seemed, she was dying for certain. It soon looked as though Jan and Barbara were going to die within the same week, possibly even on the same day.

Jan died. For a week Evon kept that knowledge from Barbara, who was in critical condition but hanging on. During the second week Barbara rallied slightly. She asked about Jan and was told the truth.

Eventually Barbara improved again, as she often had. After a long stay, the hospital told Barbara and her parents that she would either have to go to a nursing home or be discharged. Though still breathing through an oxygen tube, Barbara went home to be in the care of her mother. There she stayed in the same condition for some months. Her illness had now lingered for almost a decade.

One Sunday afternoon Barbara was praying and talking with two friends visiting from church. A voice spoke to her, and she sensed a "presence" in the room. She was told that the Lord had decided to heal her.

Barbara took off her oxygen apparatus and started to get out of bed. The one friend was a physical therapist and said, "You can't do this. You can't get out of bed." She did.

She stood beside the bed, feet flat on the floor—which was absolutely impossible. Her first impression was, "Call my dad and mom." Then she realized, "I don't need to call! I can walk out to them."

She walked out of her room and called to her folks. Her dad came first, thinking that it was her sister who called. After all, Barbara was on a respirator and had a tracheotomy, so she couldn't have sounded like that.

Next came her mother. She dropped to her knees in wonder, and reached out to touch Barbara's calves. "You've got calves on your legs!" And indeed she did.

That afternoon she walked outside, on the grass, in her bare feet. She remembers it felt so good. That afternoon she also rode in the car—on a truly joyous ride, and visited a nurse friend.

And that evening, as she walked into the church, at first no one recognized her—it had been years since Barbara had been to church. The pastor looked up in surprise, then took a step back. "That's nice," he smiled. "That's very nice." Then, overcoming his surprise, he announced, "We have a guest of honor."

The meeting became electric as people realized what they were seeing. What a great praise and testimony meeting followed! There are not many specific services that I regret missing, but I sure wish I'd been at my mother's church that Sunday night. Even talking about it still gives me chills.

It Was a Miracle

What Barbara did was impossible. Not even a healthy person can lie in bed for a week or two and then walk immediately. Barbara had been bedridden for months and seriously ill for years. Her therapist friend was right; it was physically impossible for her to stand up and walk after that long a time of immobility without passing out. Furthermore, her feet and ankles were deformed and her legs were shriveled and could not hold her up. What Barbara did completely defied medical science! It could not happen, but it did. It was a miracle!

The next week, Barbara sought out her physicians. They thought it was a temporary remission and didn't believe she was cured. The surgeon who had disconnected her bowel refused to reconnect it, because he knew he was going to have to do it all over again when she had another relapse. Barbara finally found a Christian physician who would believe that she was cured and who would reconnect her bowel.

Barbara has had no trouble since that time. She went on to school and became an operating room technician; what an exciting moment it was for me to scrub with my

ex-patient. Barbara now leads a healthy, full, and productive life.

What happened to these two young Christian
friends? Both Barbara and Jan belonged to evangelical, Bible-believing churches. Both had ministers
who believe that God can heal. Both had parents who
believe God can heal. Both had supportive congregations and families praying for their healing. Both
sought out the best medical care available—and both
failed to respond to it. Both went home to die—and
one of them did.

Hard Questions

As a physician, I can give a scientific explanation
for Jan's death; as a Christian, I can't tell you why she
died. As a believer in an omnipotent and omniscient
God, I can tell you why Barbara was healed, yet from
a scientific basis I can't explain it.

To the atheist or the non-believer, sickness or
death is just something that happens. It's bad luck,
bad genetics, or just a statistical probability. But for
the Christian, the issue is more complicated. We
have to deal not only with the illness and loss, we
have to struggle with our faith as well. Our minds
are filled with questions:

• Why is God doing this to me?
• Am I being punished?
• If I truly believe God can heal me, why should I
  need to see a doctor?
• Should I go to a "healing service"?
• Are my friends going to think I'm a sinner?
• How do I pray?

- Don't I have enough faith?
- Why doesn't God heal me?

My goal for this book is to help you deal with these questions in a practical way, so that you can better understand your illness or help your loved ones deal with theirs.

2

Healing in Scripture

At the time of Christ, there was a pool in Jerusalem that was said to have healing properties. From time to time an angel moved the waters of this pool; then the first person to get into the water would be healed. When Jesus came walking up to the Bethesda pool with his disciples one Sabbath, he was apparently not recognized, for there is no description of a clamor among all the blind and the paralyzed and the lame around the pool (John 5:2-9).

There Jesus spoke with a man who had been paralyzed for thirty-eight years and asked him if he wanted to be healed. The man said he had no one to take him into the pool when the angel moved the water. And Jesus said to the man, "Take up your bed and walk." The paralytic did so, and was instantly healed. What a spectacular miracle—a man paralyzed for thirty-eight years, walking immediately on restored legs!

But why this one man among all the lame, blind, and paralyzed gathered there? There is no indication that this man called out to Christ or demonstrated great faith. In fact, he complained that he had no friends to throw him into the water when it was moving. Yet he was singled out.

Jesus could have healed the whole lot of them with a wave of His hand. Why didn't He?

The Miracles of Jesus

We can't really discuss health and healing without first looking at Christ's healing miracles. Why He didn't heal all the other invalids at the Bethesda pool is just one of the questions raised when we look into Scripture to see how, when, and whom Jesus healed.

As a physician, I find it interesting to look at all the particular disease processes that Christ healed. To a varying extent, medical treatment is available for all of them now, whereas it was not available at the time of Christ.

Two people healed by Christ, the official's son in John 4:46-50 and Peter's mother-in-law in Matthew 8:14-15, were ill of fevers. Today many good, effective treatments are available.

In Mark 5:25-30 we hear of the woman who had been bleeding for twelve years. When she touched Christ's garment, she was healed. Today her ailment is routinely and easily treated.

Orthopedic deformities and curvature of the spine (see Matthew 12:9-13 and Luke 13:10-13) can be imperfectly treated with modern orthopedic surgery.

Leprosy now can be basically cured and prevented, though it is much more a socioeconomic disease than a contagious disease. That's because effective antibiotics will virtually cure the problem if the poverty and poor nutrition are well treated.

Speech impediments and paralysis of various sorts can be at times treated, but imperfectly. Many forms of blindness are treatable with modern surgical techniques.

So, for most of the categories of illness that Christ treated, we offer some medical help. Depending upon the illness, some treatments are more effective than others, but in Christ's time there was no treatment available for any of these entities. He clearly demonstrated that He had mastery over any disease process that existed. And he clearly demonstrated his mastery over death.

Help My Unbelief

In some circles of Christians, if someone is not healed, it is commonly considered a result of their lack of faith. Yet on several occasions in Scripture, people admitted to lack of faith and Christ still healed them.

The most graphic example is in Mark 9:14-29, where the apostles were incapable of healing the boy with seizure disorders and demon possession. The father of the boy boldly said, "I do believe: help me overcome my unbelief." And Christ healed the boy. When the apostles asked Him why they were incapable of doing it, Jesus said, "This kind can come out only by prayer." The implication of this very strong statement is that the apostles' failure to heal the boy was due to the inadequacy of *their* prayer. The problem was the healer's lack of faith rather than the sick person's. At no point was anyone who was struggling with faith not healed because of a "lack of faith."

This is entirely different from the occasions where Christ did not do any miracles because of a lack of faith. Where there was total unbelief, miraculous healing did not occur. But a struggle to believe on the part of someone in need of healing did not deter that person from being healed.

All Knowing, All Powerful

Jesus demonstrated on numerous occasions that He knew about someone who was ill or dying, even though the person was not present. In the case of the centurion's servant, Christ demonstrated His power over nature and illness by not having to be present to perform the miracle. He said words to the centurion, and someone was healed a great distance away. Christ did not have to be physically present to heal.

Jesus also demonstrated that He knew the outcome of illness. He told his disciples that Lazarus was going to die before it happened. He told the centurion that his slave was going to be healed.

In none of Jesus' miracles was there any "partial healing." The lepers are the perfect example, because to be declared clean and permitted back into society, they had to have lost all of the physical disfigurements of leprosy.

Mud, Spit, And Fingers

I'm intrigued by the stories in which Christ applied mud and spit to people and then instructed them to go wash it off in certain pools (Mark 8:22-26, John 9:1-7). No matter what you say, having someone spit in the dirt and then put the mud on you is a disgusting thing. To be told to leave it on and go some place special to wash it off sounds even more bizarre. But Jesus apparently required this as a tangible demonstration of belief.

I also notice, when reading about the healing miracles, that on many occasions Christ touched the person whom He was healing. Christ knew the power of touch. Today, after a few decades of high tech—low touch medicine, we are once more discovering the wonders of "touch."

The most spectacular instance of touch is in Matthew 8:2-4: "A man with leprosy came up before Him and said, 'Lord, if you are willing, you can make me clean.' Jesus reached out His hand and touched the man. . . . Immediately he was cured of his leprosy."

The reason this is spectacular is not only the physical miracle that occurred—a man instantly cured of all the stigmata and facial and orthopedic evidences of leprosy—but the social miracle created. To touch a leper was an absolute forbidden act in Jewish society. Lepers were unclean. Jesus was not revealing some superhuman immunity; He was demonstrating His knowledge that touching lepers does not cause leprosy while at the same time breaking down the barrier toward the sick.

I believe that Christ touched people when He was ministering to them to demonstrate that it is safe to touch people who are ill. Virtually no disease is contagious from touching, and touch is potent medicine.

Taste of Things to Come

Scripture rarely gives us any *reasons* for the illnesses or disabilities these people had. One exception is the story of the blind beggar at the pool of Saloam who was, Jesus said, blind so that he could be healed for the glory of God. It's important to notice that none of these illnesses that Jesus treated were punishment for sinful behavior. None of them resulted from the failure to follow God's "good health guidelines," which we'll discuss in detail in Chapter 5. None of the paralytics were paralyzed because of dumb things they had done. The only "lessons" to be learned from these illnesses, and the only "good" that came from them, were that the individuals were healed and Christ was firmly established to be who He said He was—the Son of God, who had mastery over illness and death. This is one of the major reasons for healing by Jesus—to certify that He is God. Perhaps, too, healing miracles give us a little taste of what heaven will be like, since there will be no imperfections and bodies will be restored to full health .

The Miracles of the Apostles

Peter, Philip, and Paul are all recorded as having done miraculous healing. They cured a paralytic and people with infections, and both Peter and Paul even raised the dead. In Acts 28:7-8, Paul treated Publius, the father of an official on an island, and "cured all of the sick."

Acts 19:11-12 says that God did extraordinary miracles through Paul so that even handkerchiefs were touched and taken to the sick, whose illnesses were cured and evil spirits driven out. I've often been skeptical about the healing effect of various ancient artifacts, but that's the implication of Acts 19:11-12. At times, ancient artifacts may very well have had some healing potential.

More Questions

In Acts 14:8-13, Paul and Barnabas healed a man who was crippled in his feet. This man, who had been affected by polio or clubbed feet or whatever, had been disabled for years. He was instantly and miraculously healed by Paul's invoking the name of Jesus Christ.

We would expect that God would use such a miracle to bring people to Himself, but this miraculous healing at Lystra did not help the apostles convince the pagans there. Instead, the people began to worship Paul and Barnabas as if they were God. In great anguish, Paul and Barnabas tore their clothes and fled the city.

Not only are we not given reasons for all illnesses recorded in Scripture, sometimes we can't even perceive the reason for the healing!

No Formula

In I Timothy 5:23, Paul admonishes Timothy to "take a little wine for his stomach's sake." This is Paul speaking—Paul who healed all the sick on an island, Paul who raised the dead, Paul who had as much faith in the power of God and the name of Jesus Christ as any man alive.

And what did Paul say to Timothy? He didn't chastise Timothy for his lack of faith regarding his stomach. He didn't tell him, "If you get right with the Lord, your stomach will be fine." And he didn't wave his hand and heal Timothy's stomach. Instead, he suggested tangible, practical treatment for it. He told Timothy, "Take medicine for your stomach. Don't be silly, treat yourself."

In II Timothy 4:20, Paul states that he left Trophimus ill in Miletus. He didn't say that because of his lack of faith, Trophimus was ill. And again, he didn't heal Trophimus himself.

Why didn't Paul heal Timothy? Why didn't he heal Trophimus? He certainly had demonstrated the ability to heal serious illnesses. He had even raised the dead. Paul was a healer. Paul had faith. Yet two of his closest associates and companions, his beloved Timothy and his co-worker Trophimus, were suffering, and Paul didn't heal them! Why? Paul, like Jesus, didn't always heal those around him.

I can't tell you why. Looking into Scripture doesn't give me any formula for "figuring out" God's healing, then or now. As a physician, it is clear to me that, today as in New Testament times, not all sick Christians get better. Some of them stay sick. Some of them continue to suffer. And some of them die.

Time and time again, I can only return to Paul's words in I Corinthians13: "For we know in part and we prophesy in part, but when perfection comes, the imperfect disappears. . . . Now we see but a poor reflection; then we shall see face to face" (vv. 9, 10, 12).

3

No One to Blame But —

It was winter, 1963. In my trusty VW bug, I was driving back to Houghton College in upstate New York on I–90, the interstate in Pennsylvania. The stretch just south of Lake Erie was a notorious snow belt. It was dark and, true to form, near-blizzard conditions. The righthand lane was plowed and there was reasonably good traction. The passing lane had been plowed but it had snowed since; there were only one or two tire tracks running through it. Ahead of me a semitrailer truck was doing 45 in a 65 mph zone.

I was young and indestructible. I was also tired. I felt I could safely do 50, maybe 53—certainly a few miles an hour more than 45 anyhow. So I pulled into the passing lane. I swerved a bit but was able to reach 65 and began to pass the truck. The road was slippery and visibility poor, and halfway through the maneuver I knew this was stupid. Nevertheless, I sped on. Somehow, I got past the truck and tried to pull back into the righthand lane. Suddenly the VW spun 180 degrees, and I found myself looking directly at the truck's headlights! I heard the blast of the truck's air horn and thought, "He can't stop!" I didn't even have time to cry out in prayer. The spin continued. In a few brief seconds (probably milliseconds) that had the drawn-out quality of a dream, my car turned a full 360 degrees in front of that semi—and kept on going. The semi slowed somewhat and then kept going as well.

My first sane thought when my heart had stopped pounding was that I felt sorry for the truck driver. I knew I had scared him to death. He had probably known all along what was going to happen and found himself helpless as the frightening scenario played out. Needless to say, I learned my lesson. I believe I am a better driver because of this experience—and I try to avoid driving in snowstorms completely. I believe God watched out for me on that winter night in 1963. I also believe if I continued to drive the same way in snowstorms, I couldn't count on His protection continuing!

Why Do We Get Sick?

Most of us believe that if we fell out a third-story window, God could protect us from being injured. At the same time, most of us also believe that if we *jumped* out of a third-story window, we would likely be killed or at least severely injured. Yet, many of our lifestyle habits are analogous to jumping out windows and demanding that God's angels keep us from getting hurt.

So when we ask the question of why people get sick or disabled, one obvious response is "because of their own poor choices." But before we look more closely at this answer, let's acknowledge the many situations where our choices are *not* to blame for our illnesses.

Because of Adam

We must begin with the sad truth of living in a fallen world: all of us have mortal bodies that are slowly wearing out and aging. Most males reach their peak of physical performance at age twenty one. For women, the peak age is about nineteen. After that, it's slowly and steadily downhill.

For example, an extensive study of cancer in males was done by Dr. Charles Huggins, winner of a Nobel prize for medicine, at the University of Chicago. Dr. Huggins said that if all men lived long enough, every one of them would develop cancer of the prostate. In his opinion, this cancer is simply the natural order of things.

Some of us, because of our genetic makeup, age more slowly than others, but none of us lives forever. II Samuel 14:14 says, "Like water spilled on the ground, which cannot be recovered, so we must die." And illness is often the natural way for death to come sooner as opposed to later. No one has been promised freedom from bodily death.

What about the deaths of infants and children? In this case illness cannot be blamed on a "wearing out body," but comes for what seems to be no reason at all. The fact of the matter is, people have searched for centuries to explain the deaths of innocent people, and no explanations exist. There are times when illness and death simply come, and God never gives us the "why." I'm reminded of the story of Job in Scripture. He suffered boils, illness, the loss of his possessions, misery, depression, and the death of his children, and at no point was he informed of why all this happened.

Because of Us

It is in the first category, that of the illnesses caused by our choices, where we are most easily able to identify some reasons for being sick. The focus of this chapter is on illnesses that are "our own fault," resulting from the lifestyle we have adopted.

One out of every three Americans dies earlier than he or she should. We get sick because of the things that we do to ourselves—the foods we eat, the things we drink, the work and play we do. The areas we'll look into in some detail include diet, alcohol, sexual behavior, pollution, stress, and "dumb choices."

Your response to what I have to say may range from shouting amen at my preachin' to getting angry at my meddlin', depending on where you find your choices lining up. But all of these examples must be considered, for they are all factors in understanding why a third of us are "dying earlier than we should."

The Supermarket Diet

What we eat and drink affects—in fact, causes—most of the major health concerns of our age. Our number one concern is weight. As a nation we are fat and getting fatter. The top ten best sellers always include at least one diet book. You can't pick up a Sunday supplement magazine without finding at least one new diet or weight reduction article. There are whole aisles of our supermarkets devoted to diet food. We have shelves of diet soda and light beer and wine. But in spite of our low-cal mania, we continue to grow fatter as a nation.

Three Problems

There are three factors about the supermarket diet that lead to obesity. The first clearly is fat. Over the past fifty years, the amount of fat in our diet has gone up significantly. It is almost impossible to go into a restaurant and have a low-fat meal. Our palate has become accustomed to and demands fat.

The second problem with our diet is one you probably couldn't guess—it's variety. We have such an abundance of food to choose from that we never get bored. You can feed people almost anything and they won't get fat on it, if that is the only food they get. People don't get fat on boring diets.

It was thought for a long time that rats and mice "had more self-control" than humans because they never got fat. They ate just the right amount, never more. But pet owners know that if you feed a dog from the table, rather than keeping it on a chow diet, it will get fat. Obesity experts found that the same is true of rats and mice. Given an unlimited "supermarket diet," the rats and mice that are normally lean will double or triple their weight in no time. The explanation is clearly in the diet, and is not that rats and mice are more disciplined than people!

The best example of people on a "chow diet" that comes to my mind is the children of Israel eating manna in the wilderness. In Sunday school it was always pointed out that God's people were ungrateful for complaining about their steady diet of manna. But any of us who have ever greeted leftovers with with an "Oh, Mom, not this stuff, again!" shouldn't cast stones at the Israelites! In any case, nutritional scientists anywhere would agree that if you put people on a well-balanced chow, combined with all the water they need, and have them walk daily, you'll end up with a healthy group of people. At the end of those forty years, that second generation of Israelites must have been a "lean, mean, fighting machine."

The third and least important problem with the supermarket diet is sugar. Most Americans mistakenly think that simple sugars and other sweets make up our chief dietary "sin." In reality, most people could leave an unlimited supply of candy bars out for snacking and not have a significant weight problem. The catch, of course, is that they must all be the *same kind* of candy bar—remember the boredom factor!

Fat of the Land

Statisticians, public health experts, and epidemiologists (experts who study the causes of disease) now have the statistical measure to demonstrate how weight affects our health. For every pound that you are overweight, there is a fairly accurate estimate of how much time that pound will cost you. That's a fancy way of saying that every pound of overweight is going to shorten your life. (One problem in studying health, diet, and culture is that cigarette smokers tend to have lower weight. Also, people who are dying of cancer have lower weight. Until statisticians were able to control for these two groups in their surveys, weight chart statistics didn't prove anything. Now it is clear that every pound of excess fat is bad.)

In the United States it is far easier to cure cancer than it is to cure obesity. Throughout history the obese people in other civilizations were the ruling class and the very wealthy; the workers were lean and even underweight. We may be the first culture where obesity is a sign of the affluence of the whole country rather than a sign of individual wealth.

Most of us are concerned about how weight affects the way we look, but that's only a small part of the problem. Being overweight has direct effects upon our health.

As a Cause of Cancer

The number one cancer in women, and one of the leading causes of death in young women, is breast cancer. While there is much yet to be learned about breast cancer, one fact is clear: the more overweight you are, the more likely you are to develop breast cancer. In fact, all of the cancers specific to females are more common in overweight women. Why is this?

The main sources of estrogen, the primary female hormone, are the female sex organs, the ovaries. Estrogen is also manufactured in fat to a small degree; thus, fatter women tend to have higher estrogen levels. All of the female cancers are estrogen sensitive. The higher the estrogen level, the more likely you are to develop one of these cancers. So, losing body fat decreases your risk of cancer. But of course this is a two-edged sword, because women need a certain amount of fat (about 10% more than men) to hormonally function as women. It is *excess* fat that they don't need.

Of course, another problem we're seeing in young women who have carried this fear of obesity too far is that they develop all kinds of hormonal problems caused by anorexia nervosa and bulimia.

Our high fat and low fiber diet also leads to other forms of cancer, especially colon and intestinal cancers. This is true in both men and women. Cultures that have high carbohydrate, low fat diets and eat natural grains have virtually no colon cancers or cancers of the intestinal tracts.

As a Cause of Heart Disease and Stroke

Cancer isn't the only price that we pay for our diet. The number one killer in the United States is heart disease and high blood pressure. Nowhere in the study of disease are the effects of diet more obvious. There is a strong correlation between the increase in heart disease and the change in our diet away from grain and carbohydrates to fat. The amount of fat in our diet and the degree to which we are overweight affects our bodies' cholesterol, which is an internal measurement of certain types of fat in our bloodstream. As we gain weight and increase the amount of fat in our diet, our cholesterol levels go up.

Basically there are two types of cholesterol, one good and one bad. A good cholesterol is HDL, or High Density Lipoprotein. The bad cholesterol is LDL, or Low Density Lipoprotein. LDL leads to hardening of the arteries, arterial sclerosis, and atherosclerosis, eventually blocking arteries and leading to coronary artery disease and heart attack, high blood pressure, and stroke.

Then, if you add high salt content to our diet—and we do—it puts added stress on the kidneys, which leads to high blood pressure. The higher the blood pressure is, the harder the heart has to work; the harder the heart has to work, the more likely one is to have a heart attack. The combination of high blood pressure and hard, narrow arteries adds strain on the heart; combined with narrowed pipes for blood vessels in the brain it can lead to strokes from poor circulation.

As a Cause of Diabetes

The more overweight you are, the more likely you are to develop what is called adult onset diabetes. Many overweight adults would not even have diabetes if they could get their weight back down to normal. The higher the weight, the more difficult it is to control the diabetes, and the higher the blood sugars go. The higher the blood sugar and the more out of control the diabetes is, the more likely one is to develop the complications of diabetes. One of the most feared complications, and one of the most difficult to treat, is diabetic retinopathy, which can lead to untreatable blindness. Other complications of diabetes are kidney failure and loss of circulation to the feet, leading to gangrene and sores. And one of the most painful complications is diabetic neuropathy, an effect on the nerves which can lead to incurable pain.

More Risks of Obesity

Much of my practice in sports medicine and fitness relates to athletic injuries of the knee. But since sports medicine now includes the treatment of knee disorders of anybody who wants to walk, I have had the opportunity to treat many overweight people with knee problems. I have personally become convinced that if one is markedly overweight (especially if female), and develops a bad knee joint for any reason, the disabling knee pain is virtually incurable. I can think of several women in my practice with this disability. Some underwent "technically successful surgery," all of them did every bit of physical therapy we asked of them, but they have remained disabled and crippled by their knee pain. The only thing they didn't do is lose weight.

What is true of knee pain and obesity is true of almost all other surgical and medical problems. If you are overweight, the chances of complications developing in the hospital are much greater. Your risks of surgery are markedly increased, no matter what the surgery is for. The more overweight you are, the more likely you are to develop a wound infection, the more likely your incision is not to heal quickly, the more likely you are to develop blood clots, phlebitis, or pneumonia, and the more likely you are to die, even from benign elective surgery. There isn't a surgeon in the world that will tell you you don't have a higher risk of complications for any treatment. If you are hospitalized for any cause or put on bed rest for any disease, your risk of sudden death increases if you are markedly overweight.

One More Problem

One of the subtle but very real effects of our diet when we changed from the farming diet of the last century, with its high grains and high carbohydrates, to the fatty diet we have today is the development of constipation. While at first glance this would seem to be a relatively minor disturbance, the problems of chronic constipation cannot be minimized. When we switched from a high fiber, high grain diet to a high fat diet, we decreased the bulk in our stools that prevented constipation.

The problems of chronic constipation develop slowly, but they are very real. The most common ailment is hemorrhoids. The repeated straining to pass hard stools leads to chronic swelling of the hemorrhoidal veins in and around and protruding out of the rectum and anus—that's what hemorrhoids are.

But it isn't simply a chronic, painful, "benign" condition. Chronic straining at toilet can lead to a swelling in the pelvic veins, which leads to increased pressure in the veins of the legs. This in turn leads to varicose veins and problems with the valves in the veins of the legs, causing sluggish and poor circulation in the veins of the legs and the pelvis. And this is one of the most common causes of phlebitis, or painful swelling and blood clots in the legs. If a clot forms before the pain and swelling develop, just from straining at the stool, you could "break the clot free" from the leg and, by bearing down, push the clot up the veins from the legs and pelvis to the lungs, causing a "pulmonary embolism" or fatal blood clot. All from the "minor" disturbances caused by a high fat, low fiber diet.

The Cost of Alcohol Abuse

The one essential ingredient for survival is water. We can go days and weeks without food but, depending on the temperature, our activity, and whether or not we're acclimated to heat, we can go only hours or possibly a few days without water. Yet water is no longer our most common drink. Our primary sources of water are soda pop, juices, . . . and alcohol.

Alcoholism and alcohol abuse are still this nation's number one substance abuse problem. About ten percent of all Americans have a physical weakness and inability to "handle alcohol." One drink of alcohol, be it beer, wine, or other liquor, will start them on the road to alcoholism or lead to repeated drunken binges. There is still more time lost to American industry from alcoholism than any other form of illness.

Recent research indicates that even a few drinks of alcohol may do permanent damage to a few brain cells, and the more you drink the more cells are permanently damaged. Alcohol also damages the liver and, over a period of years, will lead to the development of liver cirrhosis and its complications, which can cause an early death.

Drinking and Driving

Alcohol affects coordination and judgment; this is the reason alcohol and motor vehicles are such a lethal combination—the leading cause of death for the more than fifty thousand Americans who are killed every year in automobile accidents. But these deaths only tell part of the story. The statistics you don't hear about are the people who are maimed or injured, either temporarily or permanently, from the combination of alcohol and motor vehicles.

In over twenty years of practicing orthopedic medicine, I have treated hundreds and hundreds of teenagers who were injured in automobile accidents. Of those whose injuries required hospitalization, I can recall only a handful where alcohol was *not* involved in the accident.

Alcohol also reaps another toll in our country, and that is wife and child abuse. It is highly unusual to find abusive situations where drinking is not part of the picture. The same is true for many "crimes of passion," because the combination of alcohol and a hand gun can lead to sudden death.

A Well-Kept Secret

Much medical research and drug abuse research has been done on alcohol and the damage and harm that it causes, and many Protestant church groups have railed against the evils of alcohol. But there is one statistic that both medicine and the church have tried to ignore, because they don't know what to make of it. That is that repeated studies on alcohol intake and health seem to show and that people who take a drink or two occasionally, or even one to two drinks a day, of beer, wine or hard liquor, tend to live longer than not only those who drink three or more drinks a day, as you would expect, but also longer than teetotalers.

Most experts assume that this "quirk" in statistics relates to the fact that people who are able to use moderation in alcohol intake also use moderation in much of the rest of their lifestyle. It is likely that this accounts for their increased longevity, rather than some "beneficial" effect of a drink or two a day. The experts, medical or clerical, usually don't mention this interesting fact when talking to the public, probably because they are afraid that people will misinterpret and misuse it.

Sexual Promiscuity

"The mayor boarded up the bath houses and brothel and was threatening to brand or tattoo prostitutes. Special houses were built for the disease which struck terror into all the hearts by the rapidity of its spread and the ravages that it has made."

The quote is from Sir William Osler. The place was western Europe, and the year was 1494. The venereal disease that the Europeans had and spread through the world, virtually decimating Central and South American Indians as well as the natives of the Hawaiian Islands, was the "great pox," or syphilis. At that time syphilis was incurable because penicillin had not yet been discovered.

One Cost of Promiscuity

Until recently, the common venereal diseases were considered syphilis and gonorrhea, both of which were virtually curable by penicillin (although now we are beginning to see strains of both that don't respond to penicillin and require other, more potent, antibiotics). Many people considered this cost of promiscuity not too high a price to pay, because of the 99 percent cure rate with a simple drug.

But this usually mild venereal disease, gonorrhea, in

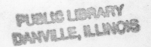

men does lead to scarring of the urethra, the passageway for urine out from the body. This can lead to difficulty in urinating and other very serious urological problems that may require surgery and are very difficult to treat.

The leading cause of infertility in women in the United States is pelvic inflammatory disease, or PID. Partly because gonorrhea is difficult to diagnose in women, and partly because of prudishness and not wanting to offend, it is the unusual doctor who will tell a woman with PID that she has probably contracted gonorrhea. Most would simply say she has an infection. But because the symptoms of pain and fever develop late in the female, there can be scarring in the fallopian tubes, causing infertility.

Other Costs of Promiscuity

Until recently, viral infections were not recognized as being transmitted as venereal disease. But two of the most serious viral infections that can be transmitted as venereal disease can also be lethal.

The latest venereal disease that has been documented to be sexually transmitted is hepatitis B, transmitted almost exclusively between heterosexuals. The principle of how you get it applies to almost all venereal diseases—as a general rule, it takes repeated sexual exposure to catch hepatitis B sexually.

If your number of lifetime sexual partners is under ten, you have no significant statistical chance of catching hepatitis sexually. However, if you have more than ten sexual partners your risk of catching hepatitis B sexually goes up dramatically. If you have more than fifty lifetime partners, the risk of catching hepatitis B quadruples.

Hepatitis B is a graphic example of the built-in

"forgiveness" or resistance that we have to sexually transmitted diseases. But the more promiscuous our lifestyle, the more likely we are to contract a sexually transmitted disease.

When AIDS was first recognized as an entity, one constant characteristic of infected males was that they all had had more than one thousand lifetime sexual partners. Initially it was a lifestyle venereal disease of homosexual males, intravenous drug users, and their sexual partners.

Living on a Fallen Planet

Pollution is bad! Pollution shortens our lives! I don't know anyone who would quarrel with those statements. Any rational person who looks objectively at how we've taken care of our planet will admit that we have not done a good job. Pollution is not only ugly, it's unhealthy and is affecting all of us. Many of the cancers that plague us are the direct result of the way we have polluted our environment, our air, our water, and our food.

In earlier times, and yet today in much of the third world, the number one public health problem is the lack of pure, clean, drinking water. And experts on ground water and pollution will tell you that much of the drinking water in the United States today is at risk of being contaminated by long-acting pollutants. These pollutants are the slow killers that cause cancer as opposed to raw sewage in third-world countries that makes you sick immediately.

There are pollutants in the food chain—pesticides that have been overused and that are now making their way into the foods we eat. Another form of pollution that we will have to deal with at some point—or if not us, then our children certainly will—is radioactive pollution. Certainly properly-channeled radioactivity can be helpful, but radioactive pollution is a dreaded and effective killer.

We have also polluted the air. Some forms of pollution we are exposed to and tolerate because of our lack of action as citizens of the earth. Other forms we are addicted to and choose willingly—like cigarette smoking, the number one killer pollutant in the United States. Non-smokers are also at risk from the secondary smoke they inhale; its effect is the same as being in Los Angeles on a smog alert day. Air pollution, whether from cigarettes, industry, or automobiles, is bad for us.

The Truth about Marlboro Men

Lung cancer used to be incredibly rare in women, but then again, so was cigarette smoking. Now that women smoke as much as men, lung cancer in women is as common as it is in men. Cigarette smoking is also implicated in cancer of the kidney, pancreas, and other organs. It cripples the lungs, leading to chronic asthma and emphysema. Cigarettes clearly shorten lives.

It's true, Scripture says absolutely nothing about cigarette smoking. However, we are exhorted to care for our bodies, and I can safely say cigarette smoking is not recommended in Scripture!

There is absolutely no question that every day you smoke cigarettes, you shorten your life. If you stop smoking, some of the damage can be undone, but not all of it. Cigarette smoking is extremely difficult to stop because nicotine is physically addicting. There is no question that nicotine is a soothing, calming drug that is immensely satisfying to its users. Withdrawal from nicotine is miserable, uncomfortable, and anxiety and stress provoking.

Most of us remember the "Marlboro man" from television commercials. He was a robust, masculine cowboy, the picture of health and a romantic outdoor lifestyle that most of us dream about. A recent TV interview showed one of the living Marlboro men. He found it painful to walk because he was so disabled and crippled with emphysema, or chronic obstructive pulmonary disease—a direct effect of cigarette smoking.

If you have ever held your breath too long under water and come up gasping for air, or run real hard in a race and in the end were "out of breath," then you can imagine what it is like to exist with emphysema. Talking is difficult. Breathing becomes almost impossible, requiring the aid of breathing machines and oxygen.

Cigarette smoking is also one of the leading causes of kidney cancer, bladder cancer, cancer of the pancreas, and lip, tongue and throat cancers. I have always said lung cancer is one of the *good* things you can get from smoking—at least it kills you quickly and gets it over with.

I used to want to be a pipe smoker because I thought it would give me a tweedy, professorial image. One rotation on the ear, nose and throat service as a medical student was all it took to cure me of that affectation. I could no longer bring myself to puff on my pipe after observing patients who had had the "Andy Gump Operation," in which the jaw and tongue and lower half of the face are removed.

A Pain in the Feet

My first year in private practice, I had a patient named Joan. She had a bad back and in fact, some years previously, someone else had done back surgery on her. She came in complaining of increasing pain in her feet, with the pain moving up to her back. She was so disabled she could not function at home. We admitted her to the hospital, but she did not improve the way a typical back patient would. In fact, it became more and more apparent that it was her feet that were "killing her."

She had peripheral vascular disease and Reynauds syndrome, that is, a hardening and spasm in the arteries leading to her feet which caused the pain. It was a result of cigarette smoking. We tried various medications; none of them gave her much relief.

She refused to quit smoking. Over a period of years we would readmit her when the pain would get out of hand. She had asked for surgery or other types of healing medications to solve the problem. It came to the point where she could barely function because of her foot pain—yet she continued to smoke. She developed gangrene in her toes, but she kept on smoking. Eventually, she had to have both of her feet amputated because of the gangrene which developed.

It is hard to imagine why anyone would willingly kill herself for the habit of cigarette smoking. But it is hard for a non-smoker to understand the addictive quality of nicotine.

Loneliness and Other Stresses of Society

Depression is the leading mental illness in the United States. Two of the major factors contributing to depression are the break-up of the family and the isolation of city and suburban life. For most people there is no longer an extended family, that support group of brothers and sisters and grandparents and uncles and aunts to talk to and confide in and lean on, but a small nuclear family consisting of husband, wife, and children—or often no family at all. And in our metropolitan "neighborhoods," it is easy to be surrounded by people and still be alone.

I worked in an emergency room in southern California in the days before paramedic mobile intensive care units. But even back in those dark ages we did have two-way radios. One afternoon the ambulance radioed the emergency room that they were bringing in a woman with a gunshot wound to the head. When they arrived, we rushed the woman into the trauma room. This was obviously a suicide attempt—and we saw at once that it would be a successful one.

There were two holes in the woman's brain, one where she held the gun to her head and the bullet entered and a much larger one on the other side where the bullet and much of her brain had blown out. She had used a large caliber pistol. Only her "brain stem" was working; she was barely breathing and her heart was functioning, but all the tests for "higher brain function" were absent.

With the woman was her purse containing a list of her family. The nurses and secretaries started calling the three names listed. The first one we were able to reach was her son. I got on the phone and told him his mother had attempted suicide and was seriously injured, and I requested that he come to the emergency room. His reply: "Oh, she's always doing that. I'm going to the beach today because the surf's up. I'm not going to waste my time coming in to see her this time." I became more graphic and told him this was not a gesture—she was probably going to die. He refused to come and hung up on me.

Next we reached her husband. I spoke with him and told him his wife was in the emergency room, had attempted suicide, and was seriously injured. He interrupted me. "Oh, she's always doing that. I'm not going to bother coming to see her this time; I've got an important golf date." As I had done with the son, I explained that this was no gesture, and if he didn't come over at once she might be dead before he got there. He refused and hung up on me.

Lastly, we reached the daughter. She, too, interrupted my speech, saying that she was on her way to a shopping mall with her friends and her mother had done this many times before. I pleaded with her to come; she refused and hung up. Within an hour, the woman was dead.

In my opinion, it was not the 44 magnum bullet that blew this woman's brains out that took her life—it was the lack of love, the isolation, and the ensuing depression that killed her.

The Cost of Divorce

Some Pharisees came to him to test him. They asked, "Is it lawful for a man to divorce his wife for any and every reason?"

"Haven't you read," he replied, "that at the beginning the Creator 'made them male and female,' and said, 'For this reason a man will leave his father and mother and be united to his wife, and the two will become one flesh'? So they are no longer two, but one. Therefore what God has joined together, let man not separate." "Why then," they asked, "did Moses command that a man give his wife a certificate of divorce and send her away?"

Jesus replied, "Moses permitted you to divorce

your wives because your hearts were hard. But it was not this way from the beginning. I tell you that anyone who divorces his wife, except for marital unfaithfulness, and marries another woman commits adultery" (Matthew 19:3-9).

It is true that divorce is extremely painful and stressful for a woman. Typically, she will be sick and have multiple maladies for a year or two. During that first year, there is a strong possibility of her being promiscuous. After a couple of years, however, the woman settles down and usually adapts fairly well without any other physical price. It is assumed that one other reason for this is the strong support network of friends that many women have. Women, in general, do share one another's burdens. They talk to each other, console each other, and generally help each other out.

Men typically seem to find the divorce process less wrenching and aren't physically affected by it as much during that first year or two. However, the single divorced man has a very shortened life expectancy. He usually has much less of a support system than his ex-wife, and the stress of loneliness and depression takes an enormous physical toll in later years if he remains single. Television, movies, books, and magazines have glamorized the single male's existence. In truth, his is a lonely, unhealthy existence.

Can a man scoop fire into his lap without his clothes being burned? Can a man walk on hot coals without his feet being scorched? So is he who sleeps with another man's wife; no one who touches her will go unpunished.
Men do not despise a thief if he steals to satisfy his

hunger when he is starving. Yet if he is caught, he must pay sevenfold, though it cost him all the wealth of his house. But a man who commits adultery lacks judgment; whoever does so destroys himself. Blows and disgrace are his lot, and his shame will never be wiped away; for jealousy arouses a husband's fury, and he will show no mercy when he takes revenge. He will not accept any compensation; he will refuse the bribe, however great it is" (Proverbs 6:27-35).

Chastity and the sanctity of married life and maintenance of family are all necessary for sound physical and mental health. That's what God wants of us. If we don't do what he wants, we do pay a physical price.

The Cost of Stress

Every year or so a popular magazine will come out with a list titled something like "One Hundred Major Stressors in Our Lives." Point values are assigned to major life-affecting events such as the death of a spouse, divorce, major sickness, loss of a job, moving to a different city, changing schools, etc. If you have a low score, you live a rather stress–free life. If you have a very high score, the article implies that you are susceptible to a major breakdown or stress–related illness.

There is no question but that major stress-provoking events in our lives can and do make us sick—but they only account for three to five percent of the stress-related illnesses that we see in our society. The major causes of stress-related illnesses are the *little things* that bug us and eat at us—the price of baby-sitters, difficulty finding day care, frustration with cooking meals, loneliness.

Think about that roommate you didn't get along with; what were the things that got on your nerves? They are usually the little things: he picked his nose, she threw her clothes on the floor, he snored, she was too neat. The little stressors are the things that really get us. Generally, it's these little stressors that cause stress-related illnesses.

A classic example is an upper-back pain that doctors have difficulty explaining and treating. Called fibrositis syndrome, it is a pain in the upper back or neck that can be disabling and cause severe spasms. It is a totally benign disease that is almost always caused by stress. The expression, "You're a pain in the neck" graphically describes the disease—but it should probably be worded, "You're a pain in *my* neck."

Colitis, ulcers, eczema, asthma, headaches, high blood pressure and its resultant stroke, kidney failure, or heart attack—all of these are caused to a varying degree by stress. Physicians use the term "target organ." The target organ is different in each of us. For some it is blood pressure, for others it is the colon or stomach or head or skin. How we handle stress hits us in our target organ.

The more high-powered and industrialized our country has become, the more stress-related illnesses have become a problem for our population. Stress is one of the major things that makes us sick.

Count to Ten

"A fool gives full vent to his anger, but a wise man keeps himself under control" (Proverbs 29:11).

"You have heard that it was said to the people long ago, 'Do not murder, and anyone who murders will be subject to judgment.' But I tell you that anyone who is angry with his brother will be subject to judgment"

(Matthew 5:21, 22a).

We understand these verses to mean that our anger results in sinful attitudes and actions toward other people, but the word from medical science is that it won't do us any good, either! Stress may be bad for you, but anger is ten times worse. The highest blood pressure, the highest heart rate, and fiercest chemical reaction recorded in the human body all happen when we become angry. If it's the little stressors that make us sick, it's anger that kills us.

If you have high blood pressure or hardening of the arteries and you get angry, you are at major risk of heart attack or stroke, literally dropping dead in a "fit of rage." Once you let your temper get away from you, it could kill you.

Enough Is Not Enough

In any sports medicine clinic, almost all the patients are there because of choices they have made. Either they have engaged in a risky activity and were injured or they are suffering from "overuse syndrome," the most common diagnosis in sports medicine. It literally means too much of any activity—too much running, too much bicycling, too much swimming, too much aerobics, too much tennis.

The American mindset is "if some is good, more is better." That is a false philosophy. It's a lack of moderation in exercise, just as it is a lack of moderation in eating or drinking, that makes us sick. An "exerciseaholic" is even harder to treat than the workaholic or alcoholic.

"Doctor, you can tell me anything except to stop aerobics," I often hear. Or an echo from the next room is, "Doctor, just don't tell me to stop running."

Our country is rapidly being divided into two classes of people: those who don't exercise enough and those who are exercising too much. There should be a third category of people, those doing everything in moderation; but unfortunately, they are small in number. As the saying goes, "The problem with common sense is that it is not that common."

You Can't Fool Mother Nature

Many exerciseaholics like not only the way they feel, but the way they look—which is younger. By exercising they are combatting the ravages of aging; in extreme cases, they believe they are "preventing" themselves from getting older.

Often these are the most difficult patients I treat—the middle aged men who are robust, handsome, and with bodies that many a teenager would envy. But a shoulder starts to hurt when they play tennis six or seven days a week. They are losing a little strength in their bench press. A knee gets sore and swells when they run more than thirty miles a week.

The problem is that these handsome, fit men are unwilling to accept any disability whatsoever. They've always had "perfect" bodies and they just won't accept the fact that they are getting older. Furthermore, they are pushing their bodies to the limit by maintaining their terrific physiques. I can treat the major problems, but I can't restore the knee or the shoulder or the elbow back to what it once was. (I have singled out men here simply because more men seem to have this problem in my practice—but it is not a gender specific problem!)

Just Plain Dumb

Nearly every person I treat for a broken bone or smashed-up joint makes a speech on this theme: "That's the dumbest thing I ever did." "I should have known better." "I told myself this was going to happen, but I did it anyway."

Every now and then an airplane will fly out of the sky and land on an innocent person, but 99 percent of the time our injuries are the result of a foolish or risky activity.

Motorcycle Madness

I remember the man who bought his daughter a motor scooter and hopped on with her to show her how to drive. Although they weren't going even thirty-five miles per hour, he suddenly realized that she didn't know how to brake or downshift. They came upon a curb and drove right into a house, breaking both his legs. Fortunately, the daughter wasn't hurt. And there was another man who bought a motorcycle and hopped on it for the first time without any lessons. Coming around a wet turn, he slid under a street sweeper and took off one leg above the knee.

I know my bias will be unpopular with many, but I've seen too many accidents to reach any other conclusion: riding a motorcycle is asking for trouble. Whenever I'm called to the emergency room to treat a young man injured in a motorcycle accident—providing he was wearing a helmet and still has a brain that is functioning and he isn't paralyzed from the neck down—one of the first things I tell him is this. "This is God's warning to you that the next time you're injured on your motorcycle, it's going to be worse."

Invariably, all motorcycle drivers will tell you that *they* are safe; it's the "dumb car driver" that ran them off the road. And to a certain extent, they are right. I can't tell you the number of times perfectly "innocent" motorcycle riders have been clobbered by automobiles, because the car drivers are geared to be looking for cars, not motorcycles. But I've had patients in long-legged casts rig up holsters on their motorcycles for their crutches, so they can get right back on and start riding.

If riding motorcycles is dumb, drinking and riding motorcycles is suicide. I remember Tommy, the janitor at my children's grammar school. At two o'clock one morning, riding home from his favorite bar at too fast a speed, Tommy hit a bump, flew off his motorcycle, and straddled a lamp post. He split his pelvis right up the middle and tore his prostate and scrotum in half. The urologist and I were up half the night trying to put Tommy back together. He walked like a duck from then on and claimed that everything still worked. The urologist doubts that he is telling the truth.

Consider the Risks

I've lost track of the number of mothers who have asked me how they can keep their sons from getting football injuries. The only sure answer is to not let their sons play football. But if the boys are going to play football, I tell the mothers to pray for rain, lots of rain, every Friday or Saturday night. At the high school and college level, most games are played on grass, and when things are sloppy and muddy, injuries are few. This past year it rained in DuPage County almost every weekend—and it was the safest football season we've had in two decades.

Football becomes more dangerous as players get bigger and older. Pee Wee football is a fairly safe little sport. In high school football, about one out of every four players will be injured enough to miss a practice or game. In college, where the players are bigger and faster, the injury rate doubles—two out of every four players will be injured enough to miss a practice or a game. And when you get to the pros, where players are bigger and faster yet, almost four out of every four players are injured every season so that they will miss practice or a game. The injury rate is over ninety percent.

While we may pray for a safe game, the fact of the matter is that when big, strong, fast men are colliding with each other, things are going to happen. If you don't want to get hurt, don't play football.

The question really is, when we willingly put ourselves in a position where we know the risk of injury is great, week in and week out, can we count on our guardian angel to protect us? Or is that "putting God to the test," as Jesus warned us not to do (Matthew 4:7)?

Remember Baretta, the TV detective of several years back? Baretta was hip, streetwise, and a bit of a philosopher. His famous line was, "Don't do the crime if you can't pay the time." Many of the unfortunate injuries that befall us are the result of the "crimes" we choose to commit. Some are not only poor choices—they are downright stupid.

While there are other explanations for why we are sick, and we will discuss these more in chapter four, don't forget the most common explanations. The first explanation, which we have discussed here in detail, is our choices and lifestyle. Second is the fact that all of us have mortal bodies that are wearing out; illness is the natural consequence of aging. A third explanation is that there frequently *is* no good explanation. And that may be the hardest one of all to accept.

— 4 —

Why Me?

In the last chapter we identified a lot of sicknesses that we have brought upon ourselves. But certainly we are not always responsible for our illnesses, either as individuals or as a society. And when a loved one dies in a car accident or we are suddenly stricken with a serious illness, it is a natural reaction to blame God. If we don't blame Him, at least we question Him: "Why me, God? Why is this happening to me?"

Many good books have been written by philosophers and theologians about why there is illness and suffering and pain in the world. (I would recommend *The Problem of Pain* by C. S. Lewis and *Where Is God When It Hurts?* by Philip Yancey.) Some of them address the difference between God directly *causing* something and God *permitting* something to happen. In this chapter we will discuss instances of both. But in either case, God causing or God permitting, it seems that we could describe the situation as God *wanting* us to be sick. And once it's happened, we need to decide what we're going to do about it. What does it mean to us? What are we to learn from this? What could God possibly have in mind either by making it happen or by permitting it— why could God possibly *want* us to be sick?

American Paganism

These questions are further complicated for most of us because, without even realizing it, we have been subtly influenced by a philosophy pervasive in our culture; I like to call it "American paganism."

Some of its tenets go something like this: "If you have your health, you have everything." "You only go around once. Grab all the gusto you can get." "Look out for number one." It's a subtle influence, coming at us through innocent radio and television jingles. But the philosophy those commercials are selling is pagan. Their message is false.

Another component of American paganism concept is the McDonald's mentality. You know what I'm talking about; if there are more than one or two people in front of you in a fast-food line, you get edgy and complain about the "long wait." We expect instant service and instant gratification.

A third concept is reflected in the commercials of various legal firms. If you have been injured, "See us and we will get for you all of the settlement you are *entitled to*." In other words, if you have been hurt or something has happened, it has to be somebody else's fault—and that somebody has to pay dollars.

And a fourth conviction of American paganism is that everything is logical and knowable. It is in man's power to explain everything through reason alone, aided by scientific research—the philosophy that has been labeled "secular humanism." But the Bible says that we don't see the big picture, we don't see everything clearly; at times we will know imperfectly.

All of these thoughts have invaded our lives without our even noticing, and some of them are decidedly un-

Christian. These life-views cannot help but affect the way we think about and deal with illness, as we shall see in the chapters to come.

For Our Own Good

When Jacob wrestled with God (Genesis 32:22-33), he wouldn't quit until he was blessed. As a result of that encounter, Jacob sustained a dislocated hip and was crippled for the rest of his life—but he was also spiritually and physically blessed. Sometimes we have to endure suffering before receiving God's blessing.

A Different Miracle

Max was a Southern Baptist. He was traveling through Texas to speak to a congregation when his eyes began failing him. Tests showed that he had posterior cataracts in both eyes. His vision deteriorated rapidly, and soon he was unable to drive or work. He couldn't even read his Bible.

A devout Christian, Max prayed fervently for a miracle to restore his sight. He also sought out medical care. Max did not threaten or stew about what God had done to him. He began experimenting with ways to make it possible for him to read something, using oversized type on boards and certain editing devices.

Four months from the time he functionally lost his vision, he had eye surgery where lenses were implanted in one eye. This was not the miracle Max had expected, but his sight was now almost as good as before he began to lose it.

You can read Max's story not in *Guideposts*, but in *Forbes* magazine. *Forbes* magazine is no devotional book, unless your religion is capitalism. Why was

Forbes interested in Max? Because during his four months of near blindness, Max invented Kwikscan, a way of reading much faster and more efficiently. Max is now a wealthy man.

According to *Forbes*, "as with many another entrepreneur who found himself sidelined or bedridden for a time, in Max, an idea took root, one that he simply had to pursue. Despite the dictates of common sense, Max decided to continue experimenting with more efficient ways to read."

The article stated that many successful inventors got their ideas while they were sick. It did not mention that many of the great hymns of our faith were also written during times of illness, loss, and depression in the lives of their authors.

The Old Two-by-Four

There is a famous old country joke in which Ed brags to Fred about his obedient, well-behaved donkey who will do anything he says just for the asking. Fred doesn't believe that—no donkey does anything unless you prod it, poke it, and beat it. So they make a wager about Ed's obedient mule. Then they go up to the donkey.

Ed takes out a two-by-four, whacks the donkey over the head, and says, "Come here." The donkey obeys. Then Ed hooks the donkey up to a cart, whacks it over the head, and says, "Pull the cart." The donkey complies.

"Wait a minute," says Fred. "What do you mean, he obeys just by talking to him? You're beating that mule over the head with a two-by-four."

"No, I'm not," Ed replies. "I'm talking to him. The two-by-four is just to get his attention."

Unfortunately, many of us are like that old donkey. God has to hit us over the head with a two-by-four to get our attention before we listen to Him.

The Cost of Non-Stop Work

Bert was the head of a large international missions organization, and his position demanded a great deal of travel. He was a tense and driven man, but he believed in exercise—which also had to be efficient, compact, and intense. When I would treat him for various maladies, I stressed the importance of relaxing and taking time off. In fact, I told him that taking rest periods would make him serve the Lord better than non-stop work.

Finally Bert developed a joint problem that made travel very difficult. After months and months of conservative treatment, therapies and medication, Bert finally found a few days in his schedule to let me operate on him. The problem was severe, but the surgery went well. Bert should have been fine, but the first day after surgery, he was totally wiped out. The second day he wasn't much better. I suspected that he was physically and emotionally exhausted.

But he insisted that he had to be out of the hospital within two days to make another round-the-world trip. I talked to his wife, who told me that this trip was not that important. She pleaded with me to keep him in the hospital for a week; if he could miss that one trip, there would be about a month before he'd have to travel again.

I geared myself up for a confrontation and walked into Bert's room, prepared to do battle. But when I ordered him to stay in the hospital another week because I felt that he needed the physical and emotional rest, there was no battle. Bert knew I was right. We gave him a full medical evaluation to rule out the possibility of any exotic infection and to justify keeping him in the hospital. All the tests came back normal. At the end of the week, he went home a new person and made an uneventful recovery from successful orthopedic surgery.

A year and a half later, Bert dropped by to thank me for what I had done. He said that week in bed had been a watershed time in his life, especially spiritually. He has a different perspective now. While he will always be an intense and driven man, he now takes time off to be with his wife and children. He is more productive and doing more for the Lord now than ever because of his times off and his rest.

Dashed Dreams

Tom and Jerry were brothers, strong, robust, healthy, athletic, and good looking. They lived for football. Jerry was a quarterback. He had a successful high school career, but in his senior year developed elbow trouble which got to the point where he could not throw at all. He saw several orthopedic surgeons, and eventually surgery was performed; but Jerry was never able to play quarterback again. Though he went on to college and made the team as a kicker and punter—and a very good one—he went through a very bitter time and wanted to know why God would "do this to him." This was very distressing to his parents, who were devout Christians.

Tom continued to have tremendous success in football. The brothers went to the same college, where Tom became the star middle linebacker for the team. His goal was to become captain of the team and lead it on to an undefeated or possibly even a national championship season.

But near the end of his junior year, Tom injured his

knee. He never missed a game, but the knee continued to trouble him with swelling and giving way. He was elected captain of the football team for his senior year. That winter he tried to wrestle, as he had done the previous two years, but the knee began to lock and he was unable to compete. Eventually he consented to arthroscopic surgery, a relatively minor knee operation. At surgery, some torn cartilage was removed. More ominously, it was noted that he had torn the ligament on the inside of his knee, the anteriorcruciate ligament. This ligament is crucial for high performance athletics. To reconstruct the ligament would mean a year of recovery for Tom; he would have missed his entire senior season. So we decided to try to get him through with physical therapy and bracing and only do surgery if he couldn't perform.

Tom worked very, very hard on rehabilitation. His roommate was a charismatic Christian who believed firmly that God would heal everyone if he only had enough faith. Tom went to his roommate's church, and the entire congregation prayed over Tom. Everyone at that service, including Tom, was convinced he was healed.

That summer Tom had occasional insecurities in the knee, but no major problems. He had done all that was asked of him in rehab and had done it well. He had faith he would be okay for the season. Tom wore a knee brace that was custom fit to his leg—but by the second game of the season, he was unable to play on the knee at all. He consented to the ligament reconstruction on the knee and missed his entire senior year. The team had held hopes for and undefeated season and at least a conference championship, but without Tom they lost games they shouldn't have and had an average season.

This was all difficult for Tom to deal with and, in a different way, it was difficult for Jerry. Neither of them could understand why they hadn't been healed. Neither of them could understand why their careers had been ruined and their team's season wrecked.

A year and a half later, Tom's mother talked to me. These episodes had been as difficult for Tom's parents as they had been for the boys, because they were Christians and they were football fans. The loss of their boys' ability to play football was disappointing for them, and they suffered with their boys because they knew what the loss of the season meant for them. And more importantly, they had had to deal with the spiritual issues raised by the boys' questions. Why had God let this happen? Or, why did God cause it to happen?

Tom's mother told me how difficult it had been to go through these experiences with the boys, especially the stress which the lack of healing put upon their faith. However, she went on to say, she and her husband had seen enormous spiritual growth occur in both boys as a result. Both of them were now going into full-time Christian service on the mission field. God had worked it all out for their own spiritual good.

A Thorn in the Flesh

The apostle Paul had the gift of healing. In fact, articles of clothing that he touched could heal. Yet his is the best example of a failure to be healed that was for his own good.

"To keep me from becoming conceited because of the surpassingly great revelations, there was given me a thorn in my flesh, a messenger of Satan to torment me. Three times I have pleaded with the Lord to take it away from me but he said to me, 'My grace is sufficient for you, for my power is made perfect in weakness'" (II Corinthians 12:7-9).

Notice that Paul prayed diligently to be rid of the thorn in his flesh. If anyone had faith that God could heal him, it certainly was the apostle Paul. But in spite of his faith and in spite of his pleading and prayer, he was not cured of his thorn of the flesh. In fact, Paul admits that God said it was there for his own good, to keep him from becoming conceited.

Secondly, notice that the thorn, while it was there for his good, was not from God but was a messenger of Satan. Even though God *permitted* Paul to have his disability, God did not cause it.

Thirdly, not only was his lack of healing *not* from a lack of faith—I don't think anyone would really question the faith of the apostle Paul—but also it was not there for punishment for anything that he had done. In fact, he was disabled or ill *because* of his faith and his relationship with the Holy Spirit and the ministry he had.

God does not need a perfect human vessel to do his will. On the contrary, it seems that the more imperfect and disabled we are, the better we can be used. "My grace is sufficient for you for *my power is made perfect in weakness*" (II Corinthians 12:9).

A physical disability or illness may actually be the result of our spirituality and our good relationship with God rather than a punishment. And the greater our gifts, the greater the risk of vanity. To keep us from becoming conceited and for our spiritual good, God may want us disabled. Furthermore, that very disability or illness may make God better able to use us than if we were physically whole.

Locker Room Pride

Over and over again I have seen people who take pride in their athletic ability or in their appearance or in some physical attribute brought down by that source of pride where it becomes something they can no longer take pride in. It is one thing to be thankful for the blessings and abilities God has given us—physical, mental, or monetary; it is another thing to be prideful about them. While we can be immensely thankful for gifts, they are ours not from accomplishment but because they have been given to us. And God does use illness and disability to discipline us, as Proverbs 3:11-12 points out: "My son, do not despise the Lord's discipline and do not resent his rebuke, because the Lord disciplines those He loves, as a father the son he delights in."

I have a friend who takes great pride in his body. He used to brag in the locker room, only half in jest, about how great he looked and what a great body he had. He was an excellent athlete and avid tennis player. Today he is disabled with back pain, unable to play tennis and unable to do the occupation that he loved.

It is quite dangerous for us to take pride and brag about our bodies, as opposed to being thankful for the health and physical gifts we have been given. Remember another familiar verse from Proverbs, "Pride goes before destruction" (Proverbs 16:18).

Homecoming

So there are many positive things that illness may bring into our lives. It may teach us a lesson. It may help us receive God's direction for our lives. It may be prevent us from becoming proud or get rid of pride we already have. There is no denying that God sometimes does make us sick for our own good. And there's another way that illness can be a channel to good, although it may not sound good to us at first—it may be God's way of calling us home.

"Dr. Dominguez, when you're done with this operation, call Dr. Blumhagen in the emergency room. Finish the operation before you call."

Now that was an unusual request. Many times I've been called to speak to ER physicians in the midst of an operation, if there is a convenient fifteen-second break we can take. But, "Don't call until the operation is over"?

As soon as the procedure was done, I called the emergency room. My good friend Rex, head of the emergency room, got on the phone.

"It's your dad! He's had a massive coronary. The paramedics have been doing CPR from the scene to here—ten to fifteen minutes now. We can't get him going. How much more do you want us to do?"

Rex knew the answer before I said it. "Stop. Let him go."

He had a bad heart and was diabetic. He had already had four to six heart attacks but was still going strong and working in his mid-seventies. My sisters kept asking me to tell him to slow down, yet deep down they knew that was wrong. Putting Dad in a rocking chair would have been a lingering death sentence. This typical Mexican American male had worked hard all his life and didn't intend to stop. He died the way he wanted to—with his boots on, driving home from work. He pulled his car over to the side of the road and collapsed in a neighbor's front yard, two blocks from home. Although his death was sudden and unexpected, we all agreed that it was the right way for him to go home.

We have to remember that heaven is a beautiful

place. While it is tough for those left behind, the apostle Paul has said, "For me to die is gain." If we believe that, then we have to believe that even death can be "for our own good."

Granted, this is easier to accept when the dying person is seventy and has lived a full life as a devout Christian than when it is a younger person, but the principle is still the same. We don't believe what we claim, if we don't believe Paul's words that is to die is gain.

For Someone Else's Good

We have seen examples of illnesses that are for our own good. There are other times when our illnesses do us no good at all, but are for someone else's benefit. This category is very difficult for us if we have bought into American paganism, and believe "number one" is the only one worth looking out for.

Ezekiel's Lovely Wife

The first example is as difficult to comprehend as any illustration that can be given. It is from Ezekiel 24:16-21.

"Son of Dust, I am going to take away your lovely wife. Suddenly, she will die. Yet you must show no sorrow. Do not weep: let there be no tears. You may sigh, but only quietly. Let there be no wailing at her grave: don't bury your head nor feet, and don't accept the food brought to you by consoling friends."

I proclaimed this to the people in the morning and in the evening my wife died. The next morning I did all the Lord had told me to do. Then the people said, "What does all this mean? What are you trying to tell us?" And I answered, "The Lord told me to say to the people of Israel, I will destroy my lovely, beautiful temple, the strength of your nation and your sons and daughters in Judea will be slaughtered by the sword."

It is quite clear in this story that Ezekiel's lovely young wife was stricken with a fatal illness and died very quickly in one day's time, and that her death certainly did Ezekiel no good. Her illness was clearly not a punishment for anything she had done nor anything Ezekiel had done. In fact, it was because of Ezekiel's close relationship with God that this all happened. Her death was an example, an illustration to the people of Israel to whom Ezekiel was prophesying of what was going to happen. Just as Ezekiel lost his wife, God was going to lose his bride Israel suddenly and swiftly if they didn't repent.

I believe in the divine inspiration and inerrancy of the Bible, and I believe it speaks to us today as it did to people 2000 years ago. But I also recognize that Scripture was written by men with an Eastern mindset, and this makes some passages particularly difficult for us, with our Western ways of thinking, to understand and discuss. This is such a passage.

How could a loving God strike a lovely, righteous woman dead as an illustration for sinners? Worse yet, for sinners who did not repent as a result? It makes us say, "What a waste!" or, "How unfair." I suspect many of us would at the least question God's judgment if faced with the same scenario.

But the thing to notice in this example is that Ezekiel accepted this prophecy and his wife's death with a grace and understanding far greater than most of us could muster. At no point does he react with bitterness or question the decision. His behavior is a beautiful and tangible demonstration of his faith in an omniscient and all-loving God.

Preaching vs. Practicing

The closer we are to God, and the more we commune with Him, the more we see His loving nature and the superiority of His will and design above our desire or understanding. Most of us give lip service to our faith in God's omniscience and will for our lives. Yet, when that collision of faith and works occurs, when we must act or react to the tangible, painful prodding of the Lord, how we react says more about our faith than anything we profess.

As a physician and surgeon I have treated and observed thousands of Christians when they are sick, hurting, and disabled. I have watched hundreds of families struggle with serious illness and death.

Preachers talk about the interaction of faith and works; I can tell you from experience that there is no dichotomy between the two when we're hurting, sick, dying, or facing a loved one's death. Then we truly practice what we believe.

I have known professing Christians who were a joy to treat, a glorious witness in the face of suffering. I have known others who behaved in ways that seemed to me markedly unchristian. When faced with terminal illness, they behaved in ways that mocked their profession of belief in the existence of heaven or faith in a God who has power over illness and death.

For God's Glory

Another example of an illness for someone else's

good is the blind man at the pool of Siloam. "He went along, He saw a man blind from birth. His disciples asked Him, 'Rabbi, who sinned, this man or his parents, that he was born blind?' 'Neither this man nor his parents sinned,' said Jesus, 'But this happened so that the work of God might be displayed in his life'" (John 9:1-6).

Christ went on to heal the man of his blindness. But the important thing to note is that Christ categorically stated that the blindness was not the result of the man's sin nor his parents' sin, nor was it punishment. The man was blind for the glory of Christ, so that he could be a demonstration of his healing ability to the disciples.

For the Progress of His Kingdom

Nate Saint, Ed McCully, Pete Flemming, Roger Youderian, and Jim Elliot were five young men killed by gang violence. They were college educated men, most of them married, and they were missionaries in South America. The "gang" was a group of Auca Indians who had never been reached with the Gospel. At the time, the whole mission's project was in jeopardy. Five families were broken, five young men were dead. What a waste. What a loss. None of it made sense.

Twenty-five years later, evangelical churches and mission boards agree that the death of those five young men did more to encourage young people to go into missions and open up more countries to the Gospel than did any other single event in the last thirty years. The Lord's hand was in it and this event was used mightily—for the benefit of Christ's kingdom, not for the five who were dead. Jim Elliot, one of the five, stated it succinctly when he said, "He is no fool who gives up what he cannot gain to gain that which he cannot

lose." Those five men gained an "early homecoming."
And the field of missions has never been better served
than by those five deaths.

The Others Who Are Watching

If you're a Christian, others watch you. They know
the faith you really believe is the faith you practice. And
they pay particular attention to how we behave when
we are hurting or dying.

Tunis was a devout man of God, a wonderful pastor.
His last church was in Michigan, where God used him
to shepherd a fine body of believers into a thriving, vibrant church. He finally felt that it was time to retire. He
and his wife were so beloved that they were given the
parsonage to use for the rest of their days.

Perhaps one of the reasons Tunis felt called to retire
was that he was experiencing the effects of severe heart
disease. Five weeks after a heart attack, which at first appeared mild but in reality caused major damage to a
valve, he almost died one morning. Emergency open
heart surgery using valves and bypasseswas his only
chance. There was a good probability he would not survive it, but without it, he would die within hours.

His family all gathered. One son, a missionary, returned home from the field. They had a family prayer
meeting before the surgery and the family and church
friends held a vigil outside the operating room the day
of the operation.

The surgery went without a hitch. After a year he recovered well enough to want to preach. He and his wife
prayed that God would give him opportunities to share
the word—"Not too many, and not too few. Just what
my health can bear. From that Sunday on, for a complete year, he had a preaching engagement every Sun-

day. But for some strange reason, he didn't have a single event booked after the second week in January.

The Tuesday after the last scheduled speaking engagement, he went to the hospital for tests. This time, the tests showed a critical problem with the valve, and a second heart operation was cited as his only option. Further prayer was offered, and the emergency surgery was begun. But this time, the medical team could not get his blood pressure back up. The heart was failing, and Tunis was dying. It would only be a matter of a few hours.

Once again, the family gathered in the midnight hours, but this time their hope was not on recovery, but in the eternal promises of Christ. A beautiful family prayer and praise meeting was held in intensive care at the medical center, complete with scripture reading, singing and words of eternal hope. Tunis was aware of what was happening around him even though he couldn't speak because of the breathing tube. He would gesture and wink and nod in agreement; the nurses commented on his unusual alertness, because with the low blood pressure, he should have been unconscious. It was a spiritual time, a beautifully loving, caring time.

Five years later, Tunis' wife was in a shopping mall near her home. A woman stopped her and said, "I know you, you're Tunis' wife."

"Yes," she replied, "but I don't recognize you."

"I was one of the nurses who cared for Tunis in intensive care the night he died," the woman replied. "The staff still talks about him. We've seen many people die in our unit, but never anyone so beautifully! Several of us were changed by that experience."

That is a great testimony to what the death of a Christian should be like—an inspiration to others, rather than a time of defeat. But I ask a question: Why is Tunis the only one they remember? Surely he was not the first professing Christian to have died in that unit!

Many Christians pray to be used as a witness. Sometimes their prayers are answered when they become sick. They are given the chance to be a true witness of God's grace in their lives, but they lose a wonderful chance by how they react to the illness.

For Punishment

Often if we are sick, some Christians will behave differently toward us. They believe that all sickness is the result of God's judgment for sinful behavior. Of course, if you care to get philosophical, Adam's fall in the Garden of Eden brought the curse of sickness, aging, and death on us all. In that sense, all sickness is the result of sin in the world. But that is distinctly different from one individual becoming sick as a punishment for his or her sins. It is clear from Scripture that sickness and death as God's punishment is entirely different from natural occurring sickness, or even from illness that results from not following God's "good health guidelines," which we will discuss in detail in Chapter 5.

Think for a moment of a father and child. Every parent tells his child not to play with matches. If the child doesn't listen, plays with matches anyway, and gets burned, it's not the parent's fault. The parent didn't take a match and burn the child to teach him a lesson. Being burned is a *consequence* of the disobedience, not a punishment for it. It's the same as God's good health guidelines. He warns us what to do and what not to do; if we don't listen, we probably will get burned. But if a child is flagrantly disobedient, then the child will be punished. So it is with God and His church.

For Judgment from God

In II Kings 5: 26-27, Gehazi was struck instantly with leprosy because he lied to Naaman about Elisha.

In II Samuel there is the example of David and Bathsheba, whose first child was struck with an illness and died as a direct punishment for David's sin of adultery and murder of Bathsheba's husband.

In Acts 5:1-11, we find the sad story of Ananias and Sapphira. Separately they lied to their whole congregation about the amount of money they had given to the church. As a direct punishment for lying, they were struck dead.

You will notice that all my examples were from Scripture, where we see that God has used sickness and death as punishment for flagrant violation of his commands. I do not have any real life examples, because I cannot judge others. It is not my place to know if they are "right with God," or if they are being punished.

Important Points About Sickness as Punishment

There are some important points to notice about these incidents. First of all, there was no natural connection between the illness they contracted and their sin. It's the difference between a child burning himself with matches or being spanked for playing with matches. The punishment was not the natural consequence of the act.

Secondly, in each instance, the people were *told* that they were being punished for their sins by this illness. It was no secret why they were sick or killed.

Thirdly, and most importantly, in every instance where the person was told their illness was a direct punishment from God, they never recovered—even if they were forgiven. The best example of this is David. He prayed, fasted, and pleaded with God for his child's life. He certainly had faith in God's ability to restore him. And though he was forgiven for his sins of adultery and murder, and was a man "after God's own heart," the child died. This is punishment.

When contemplating sickness and death as punishment, it's important to remember these points. Illness as punishment is not the natural consequence of wrongdoing. The person being punished knows what the punishment is for. It is not subtle. Ananias and Sapphira and David and Gehazi were all told openly and publicly what their sin was and why they were being punished. And finally, forgiveness is always available, even though a person will probably still face the consequences of the illness. Remember that, while we may become sick or disabled as a *consequence* of our poor choices or wrong actions, God's use of illness as a *punishment* is incredibly rare.

"The Sin vs. the Sinner"

These thoughts have a direct bearing on how we as Christians respond to those suffering from AIDS in our land. Here is a group of sick and hurting people who are literally being cast out of their houses, fired from their jobs, ostracized, thrown out of communities, and becoming bankrupt trying to pay their bills. We condemn them from the pulpit and the newspaper. Individually, people scoff at them and literally throw stones at them. Mother Teresa had to come from India to the United States to set up shelter to feed, care for, and love American men dying of AIDS because, for the most part, the attitude this "Christian" nation has shown these men has been as unchristian as can be.

If, as some Christians proclaim, our nation is under the wrath of God because of AIDS, surely a significant portion of that wrath will be directed at us for the way we have treated these suffering people. I keep hearing Jesus' strong words from Matthew 25:44: "They also will answer, 'Lord, when did we see you hungry or thirsty or a stranger and needing clothes or sick or in prison and did not help you?' He will reply, 'I tell you the truth, whatever you did not do for the least of these, you did not do for me.'"

God's Good Health Guidelines

In August of 1987, I was invited to participate in the Cooper clinic on fitness and health. There were gathered the world's authorities on nutrition, heart disease, diet, exercise, and fitness. As a speaker, I had the opportunity to attend most of the lectures that were given as well. As the days of that conference went on, it occurred to me that the advice these experts were giving was essentially a Sunday school lesson. Their recommended lifestyle lines right up with that given by God in the Bible.

In other words, good health is the usual result of following God's decrees and rules. The Bible describes God as our Father. Just as fathers give advice to their children and hope that they will follow it, so it is with God. He wants us to follow his rules and decrees. Doing so would add twenty years of life to the average American.

Many Christians believe that God's promise and instructions to the Israelites were for a small band of people in a particular time, but I strongly believe that Exodus 15:26 speaks to all of us today: "If you listen carefully to the voice of the Lord your God and do what is right in His eyes, if you pay attention to his commands and keep all his decrees, I will not bring on you any of the diseases I brought on the Egyptians, for I am the Lord who heals you."

So if reading Chapter 3, with its long list of things we're doing wrong, got you depressed, take heart. Here's the other side of the coin: a list of things you can do to increase your chances of good health and a longer life.

Control Your Diet

"Oh, Lord, You know how exciting it is to play Russian Roulette. Don't let me blow my brains out, Lord, when I play today."

I have never heard anyone pray this prayer, but the way we eat and then pray for healing from the resultant illnesses, we might as well!

The Bible addresses diet in both the Old and New Testaments. We usually think of Leviticus 11 where the Lord names for Moses and Aaron the animals which the Israelites are not to eat, for they are "ceremonially unclean." The list includes the camel, coney, rabbit, pig, sea food without fins or scales, eagle, vulture, black vulture, red kite, black kite, raven, horned owl, screech owl, gull, hawk, little owl, cormorant, great owl, white owl, desert owl osprey, stork, heron, hoopoe, bat, all flying insects, weasle, rat, any great lizard, gecko, monitor lizard, wall lizard, skink, and chameleon! Most of us can give up all the animals on that list without difficulty, with the exception of the pig and the sea food without fins.

This same list of animals is represented in Acts 10:11-15 in the story of Peter's dream. In the dream, Peter sees all of these animals coming down from heaven on a sheet, and the Lord specifically tells Peter that he can eat them. When Peter argues that they are unclean, the Lord replies, "Don't call anything unclean that I have made."

The key words in these accounts are "ceremonially unclean." Other New Testament references make it quite clear that the Old Testament ceremonial categories of sacrifices and cleanliness no longer apply. "Eat anything sold on the market without raising questions of conscience," Paul says to the Corinthians (I Corinthians 10:25), and to Timothy, "Everything that God made is good, and nothing is to be rejected if it is received with thanksgiving" (I Timothy 4:4). The diet restrictions of Leviticus have been lifted.

Still Good Advice

Again, there are observations that I, as a physician but not a theologian, cannot help making when I read the Bible. In Genesis 1:29, God said to Adam and Eve, "I give you every seed bearing plant on the face of the earth and every tree that has fruit with seed on it."

Grains and fruits are the basics of any healthy diet. They are nutritious, high in fiber, and essentially non-fattening. A diet high in grains and fruit will help prevent cancer, heart disease, high blood pressure, and obesity, for it is almost impossible to get fat on these foodstuffs.

Later, in Genesis 9:3, God broadens our diet to include meat: "Everything that lives and moves will be food for you. Just as I gave you the green plants, I now give you everything." The exceptions, the "ceremonially unclean" animals, we have already named.

Another important guideline that leaps off the page at me is found in Leviticus 3:17: "This is a lasting ordinance for the generations to come, wherever you live: you must not eat any fat or any blood." Following this Old Testament commandment is one of the healthiest moves a twentieth century American can make.

Get the Fat Out

Any physician, epidemiologist, or public health expert will name the number one problem with the American diet as *fat*. It is the fat in our diet that is making us obese and it is the fat in our diet that is killing us.

There are two kinds of fats, saturated and unsaturated. Unsaturated fats are generally good for us. These are fats that are liquid at room temperature, such as olive oil, fish oil, and cod liver oil. It is the saturated fat in our diet that is the problem. These are basically fats that are solid at room temperature like lard, butter, thick creams, and animal fats.

Fat is the material that makes cholesterol, and it is cholesterol that coats the blood vessels and leads to narrowing and hardening of the arteries. This is the prime offender in the major medical killer that we face—heart disease and stroke.

There is so much fat in the American diet that a person whose lab report shows a "normal" cholesterol level may still be at a high risk for coronary artery disease and heart attack. You see, rather than stick with rigid standards for cholesterol, hospitals of this country have behaved a little bit like the proponents of situational ethics—most people have high cholesterol, so that must be normal. Rather than scare people, they cranked the "normal" values up. At many hospitals, the normal cholesterol levels go up to 250 or 270. Any physician, cardiologist, or nutritionist would tell you that this is an abnormally high cholesterol level and can put one in a high-risk category for heart disease. The best research shows that we all should have cholesterol below 180 to seriously reduce our risk of heart disease and stroke.

The major factor affecting our cholesterol is the amount of fat in our diet. The only effective way to lower our cholesterol level is to eat less fat; no medication and no amount of exercise will do it.

Practice Moderation

"Wine is a mocker and beer a brawler; whoever is led astray by them is not wise" (Proverbs 20:1). The leading cause of death in people under twenty-five is accidental death. The leading cause of accidental death is automobile accidents. And the leading cause of automobile accidents is drunk driving.

"Oh, Lord, you know how I like to party. I am probably going to get drunk tonight. Please protect me and get me home safely without hurting anyone on the way." That is the prayer of people who drink and drive.

As we mentioned in Chapter 3, about ten percent of the people in the United States have a genetic or congenital weakness towards alcohol. That means, if they begin to drink, they are on a greased path to alcoholism or repeated drunken binges. There are certain populations where that number clearly is higher. (Missionaries and anthropologists from Pau Pau , New Guinea, for example, report that the Aborigines there have a genetic sensitivity to alcohol. For these people, alcohol immediately leads to drunkenness.)

One of the reasons the Protestant church railed so strongly against alcohol was to protect that ten percent for whom one drink is too much. Many evangelical churches find complete abstinence from alcohol the only acceptable alternative.

Alcoholism and drunkenness is a major physical and emotional stressor in family life today. It is implicated as the leading cause in child abuse as well as wife abuse.

And of course, alcoholism is physically destructive to the drinker, as we mentioned in Chapter 3, causing damage to brain cells and to the liver. From both a medical and a Biblical perspective, the costs of excessive drinking warrant moderation, if not abstinence.

The Benefits of Fasting

I have a surgeon friend who showed up one day about thirty-five pounds lighter than he had been. He appeared to be fit and full of energy.

"Hey, you look terrific," I said. "How did you do it?"

His answer: "Ramadan."

This man is an Egyptian and practicing Muslim who follows the feast of Ramadan, a one-month fast that all Muslims must honor. It is a limited fast but is strict in one respect: they must take no food or drink during the daylight hours during the entire month of Ramadan. At night, they are permitted to eat and drink, and they do. In the Middle East, the restaurants open at sunset and the partying and feasting goes on all night.

As a physician, it is difficult to imagine how, in the hot Mideast, people are able to go without water all day long. In sports medicine, we would certainly condemn the practice of withholding water, especially in a desert situation. But fasting has not been studied extensively. Long-term starvation has been studied, but true fasting for a day has received little medical attention.

In Biblical times, fasting was recommended as a spiritual discipline. A time for prayer and meditation was almost always accompanied by fasting. We will address the spiritual benefits of this regimen later in this chapter, but for now let us simply look at the physical health benefits.

The Discipline of Fasting

We are an undisciplined people. We have convinced ourselves that we cannot be hungry. The nutritionists tell us, "Breakfast is the most important meal of the day." Our parents exhort us to clean our plates. We are told not to miss any meals. All of our training is against fasting.

But it is possible to function for a day without food and coffee (caffeine), and just take in water. We can still exercise, we can still work hard. Fasting for a day every now and then—say, one day every two or three months, or even one day a month—is a good physical discipline. I am not aware of any guidelines as to how often one should fast, but I think it is a discipline from which we all can benefit.

I am convinced that any healthy person, eighteen years or older, can function perfectly well for a twenty-four hour period of fasting from all food and nourishment except water. Your fast can be on a regular working day; it can be on a day that you exercise. I think that you will find it will not adversely affect your performance.

I do not recommend fasting for anyone with medical problems such as diabetes, or for any growing person (that means children and young teens, at least). If you decide to fast, don't use it as a justification for pigging out the day before or the day after your fast.

Fasting can teach us to get used to being hungry and not demand that we be satiated at all times. It is a good way to shed a few pounds. But the important thing is that it will get our bodies used to getting by with less at times. It will help us fight that "McDonald's mentality" that says we must be satisfied the moment we feel a tinge of hunger.

The Benefits of Biblical Standards of Sexual Behavior

"If you reject my decree and abhor my laws, and fail to carry out all my commands and so violate my covenant, then I will do this to you; I will bring upon you sudden terror, wasting diseases, and fever that will destroy your sight and drain away your life" (Leviticus 26:15-17). Change a few words, and it sounds like an anchor man reading the six o'clock news: "If you don't practice 'safe sex,' you will catch wasting diseases that will drain away your life." The public at large has discovered what the Bible has said all along: there are consequences of violating God's laws, and they may include sickness.

The sanctity of marriage and abstinence from sexual activity outside of marriage are not popular ideas in our society, yet these are the Biblical standards. "Flee from sexual immorality," writes Paul in I Corinthians 6:19. "All of the sins that man commits are outside his body, but he who sins sexually, sins against his own body."

Sexual libertarians demand the rights of "consenting adults" to be promiscuous and practice any type of sexual behavior. They don't want to hear any scriptural pronouncements against adultery or homosexuality. But the truth is, our society would not be affected with venereal diseases if we did not violate God's laws regarding sexual behavior.

Chastity and the sanctity of married life are necessary for sound physical and mental health. Some may find this stand Puritannical or unrealistic, but it is in fact a description of what is best for us. Not only is sex within a faithful marriage the ultimate in safe sex, it is the ultimate in beautiful and fulfilling sex. It is what we were designed for, and anything less just won't be as good.

It is important to remember, however, that a judgmental or unloving attitude toward other people because of any physical ailment they have suffered as a result of their behavior is decidedly unchristian. We have all committed sexual sins, when we apply the spirit of Jesus' strong words in Matthew 5:28: "I tell you that anyone who looks at a woman lustfully has already committed adultery with her in his heart." Forgiveness of sins is available to all.

The Benefit of Rest

When asked the secret of good health and fitness, an internationally known cardiologist and fitness instructor replied, "Take a nap."

The leading cause of most conditions that wreck athletic performance, and the leading cause of injury in a sports medicine clinic, is performing or training when fatigued.

I have a good friend who, in his mid-thirties, decided to take up running. In his first marathon he qualified for the Boston marathon—no small achievement. Once he realized how truly talented he was in running, he began to train and to improve.

As he increased his training, I started to see him in the office with a variety of stress fractures and overuse injuries. One thing that was immediately obvious was that whenever he ran seven days a week, he was injured. I pointed this out to him several times, yet he would continue to go back because most track coaches and most articles offer a seven-days training schedule. It was that American mindset again—the more training the better.

He continued to push, and his injuries became so severe that he was unable to run. Today, he no longer competes in marathons or road races. In fact, he can barely run two days a week for a total of six miles.

There is no research that proves training seven days a week will injure you. But I can tell you from talking to athletes for twenty years that if you train seven days a week, the chances are you will have an injury and a breakdown.

An Unpopular Commandment

During World War II, our factories were cranking up to mass produce war material. The assembly line invariably found that they got more work per week when workers worked six days and took the seventh day off than when they were worked seven days a week.

Centuries ago this "good health guideline" was laid down as a commandment: "Six days do your work, but on the seventh day do not work, so that your ox and your donkey may rest and the slave born in your household, and the alien as well, may be refreshed" (Exodus 23:12). And in Jesus' words, "Come with me by yourselves to a quiet place and get some rest" (Mark 6:31).

Sabbath is the seventh day. Sabbatarians are those who honor the Sabbath and do no work on that day. On the Sabbath, they attend church and do other relaxing things, either spending time with family or meditating, but taking a break from work (and training).

The two groups that come to mind when we speak of Sabbatarians are Orthodox Jews and Seventh Day Adventists. It is also interesting to note that for both of these strict Sabbatarians, Saturday rather than Sunday is their Sabbath. There is no question but that Orthodox Jews and Seventh Day Adventists lead healthier lifestyles that those who practice a less strict observance of the Sabbath, although it's virtually impossible to substantiate with medical studies; there are too many factors and variables involved.

If you are acquainted with an Adventist or Orthodox Jew, ask what being a strict Sabbatarian "costs" them. There are certain occupations they don't do simply because of the requirement that they work on Saturday. But you may be amazed at the profound spiritual, physical, and emotional benefits they claim to enjoy. Most of them don't see themselves as giving up anything; rather, they see honoring the Sabbath as a restful, non-stressful, relaxing, worshipful time that they wouldn't trade for anything.

A Plus for the Family

Child psychologists, educators, and advisors advocate "quality time" spent with our children. There are many recommendations and tips on how to get that quality time, but I personally believe that the term is overused. You have to spend time with your children, and if you spend enough time with them in a variety of settings, you will get some "quality time" out of it.

The beauty of being a Sabbatarian is that one day out of seven you spend time with your family, and out of that time, quality time will evolve. While the children may moan and groan about some of the restrictions they have in Sabbatarian households, as adults they will value their memories of these times they spent with their parents.

Spending one day a week with your family may force you to talk to your spouse and improve communication between you, helping to preserve your marriage.

Remember what our world famous fitness instructor said? "Take a nap." Taking a day out of seven off will give you the rest and relaxation you need to be productive. It will help you decrease the stress in your life. It will let you get a little rest and relaxation which you need. I believe that God will honor your observance of the Sabbath and bless you for it.

Stress Management

One of the latest buzz words in health and disease prevention is "stress management." Psychologists, parapsychologists, gurus, yogis, modern science and the religious community all offer approaches to relaxation .

Biofeedback is the modern psychologist's way to physically train you to relax, lower your blood pressure, and reduce the stress in your lives. It takes months of physical and mental training with a trained psychologist to learn biofeedback techniques, but the same type of physical and mental can occur from practicing the Orthodox Jesus prayer or the Catholic rosary.

The "Jesus prayer," is a classic Orthodox prayer in use from at least prior to the 13th century. One version is, "Lord Jesus, Son of God, have mercy on me." Another version is prayed: "Lord Jesus Christ, Son of God, have mercy on me, a sinner." People who use this prayer often carefully regulate their breathing to be in time with the prayer. Monks and pilgrims found the combination of prayer and timed breathing an effective way to pass the miles or to overcome cold and inclement weather.

Another way to use the Jesus prayer is to use a *hesychast* method of prayer—that is with head bowed, chin resting on the chest, and eyes fixed on the heart, breathing in and out in time with the words. This time-honored prayer is far superior to any mantra or nonsense words that you could say.

Prayer and Meditation

There's no question that regular periods of meditation are one of the secrets to stress management. While simply sitting in a relaxed posture and chanting a nonsense word or "mantra" can be very relaxing., to the believer, all these techniques are a parody of the real thing.

With the aid of the Holy Spirit, we can commune with the one true God, who created the force that is in us and who formed the earth and holds it together.

One of the most common and frequent Biblical commands is to take time for meditation and prayer. "Pray continually," was the advice of the apostle Paul (I Thessalonians 2:20). "Blessed is the man [whose] delight is in the law of the Lord ; . . . on His law he meditates day and night," said the psalmist (Psalms 1:1). But if there is anything that is neglected in modern America, it is daily prayer and meditation.

When we meditate and pray to God, we are functioning at our highest level. It isn't a chore; it is a blessed, wholesome, relaxing, fulfilling time. It is a time we shouldn't want to miss rather than a time we have to spend. And it is something that can't be rushed; there is no substitute for it. The more we do it, the better we get at it and the better it is for us.

Reaping the Physical Benefits of Meditation

While I run the risk of being overly technical by laying down rules, that doesn't mean that the facts I want to share here are incorrect. So, acknowledging the risk, let me lay out some clinical guidelines and suggestions.

It takes at least fifteen minutes a day, five times a week, to reap the physical benefits of regular meditation. Furthermore, one has to adhere to this routine for at least three months to reap these physical benefits. So if you're hoping to use regular meditation simply as a tool to aid you physically in stress management, or in solving or treating a stress related illness, it is not a quick cure! It takes months of disciplined practice to reap the physical benefits of daily meditation.

At the risk of again being overly clinical or legalistic, let me make a suggestion to those of you who do not have a prayer, meditation, or Bible study time: buy a one-year Bible! One-year Bibles are available in many different versions, including the Living Bible, King James, and the New International Version. These Bibles have various portions of Scripture from both the Old and New Testaments listed by daily passages. In a calendar year, you will have completely read through the Bible.

All of us can manage to get up fifteen minutes earlier, find a quiet place, read that day's passage, and pray. If you have read this far into this book, then you have the ability, intelligence, and self-discipline necessary to make a daily meditation and prayer time. I guarantee that if you do that daily for three months, you will be a better person both physically and spiritually.

Managing Stress

I don't mean to imply that all stress can be managed by regular prayer and meditation. It would be a cruel hoax to tell someone who is undergoing a great deal of suffering from the physical maladies of stress that, if only they "pray and get right with the Lord," they will be able to manage their stress better. When you are suffering and under stress, it is difficult to meditate and pray. To be told by Christian "brothers and sisters" that if you meditate and pray, your stress will go away, is simply like pouring gasoline on a fire to put it out.

While there is no question that regular prayer and a meditation life is good for us, it is also commanded in Scripture. It is essential for our spiritual life and it is one of the best things we can do for our mental and physical health.

"Bodily Exercise"

Most of us raised on the King James version of the Bible can quote Paul's statement that "bodily exercise profiteth little" (I Timothy 4:8). Theologians agree that the exercises spoken of are really *religious* exercises, such as beating yourself with thorns or crawling up cathedral stairs. Those types of "exercises" profit little.

But why doesn't the Bible address exercise and fitness? I believe the answer is that it wasn't an issue for any of the people for whom it was written at that time. In a culture where people walk everywhere they go, physical fitness is a given. The writers of Scripture couldn't have envisioned a society where people rode everywhere sitting down—and in conveyances that required no effort at all.

The automobile, while a boom to our society, is a bane to our bodies. First of all, it deprives us of exercise. The hours we spend riding in an automobile let our muscles atrophy. Secondly, bouncing around in a automobile gives our bodies "microtrauma," a fancy word for injuries that every little bounce causes. Added up over a period of hours, days, and years, these microscopic injuries lead to back and neck pain. Thirdly, the automobile is a prime polluter of the air we breathe, a leading cause of lead poisoning and a host of other lung problems.

Emotional Benefits of Bodily Exercise

Our bodies were designed to work hard and to exercise. We get tougher and stronger in muscle, organ function, and bones if we exercise. Without exercise, our bones soften and become osteoperotic; our muscles atrophy and get weak and we sag and get pot bellies; our blood pressure goes up; weakening and atrophying of leg muscles puts more strain on our heart, leading to heart disease.

In addition, there are beneficial emotional effects of exercise. Lack of exercise causes anxiety and depression. One of the best physical ways to handle anxiety and depression is to get on a regular exercise program.

So to gain that twenty years from our Biblical lifestyle, we have to exercise regularly. Actually, all the exercise we need for fitness and good health is walking. All it takes is thirty minutes of *continuous exercise* three days a week to reap these physical and emotional benefits, and walking is the easiest and safest way to get it. You can also swim, bike, run, ski, or do aerobics, as long as it is non-stop exercise.

For weight reduction and weight loss, low-intensity, long bouts of exercise such as walking are far better than short bursts of intense exercise such as hard running or running up stairs, etc.

To get the most out of our bodies, to be successful, to be productive, to be creative, we must use our bodies physically as well as mentally and spiritually and socially. If we don't, we pay the price, and one of the prices is ill health.

If you follow God's good health guidelines, you are on track for physical and spiritual health. And you can't separate the physical from the spiritual, because we are spiritual as well as physical beings. To be truly healthy, we have to have a sound mind and a sound body. God wants us to have both. And to have both, we have to follow His guidelines.

6

Getting the Most From Traditional Medicine

Good health guidelines are great. It's terrific to know that, if we follow them, we've increased our chances of a long and healthy life. But the reality is that some people, including some Christians, will get sick anyway. We've discussed a number of reasons why that may happen, and admitted that there may not be any reason that we can ascertain. So if you do become sick or disabled, what then? How do you go about getting better?

First you must be sure you're getting all you can from traditional medicine. And how do you do that? By carefully choosing a doctor, by knowing how to talk to him,* by knowing when to seek a second opinion, and by understanding the strengths and weaknesses of modern medicine.

---

*Please do not interpret my referring to the physician as "he" or "him" as a bias against female physicians; rather, it is a bias against the clumsiness of "he/she" writing. When I attended medical school, male students outnumbered females by more than ten to one, and men are still the majority of practicing physicians. Fortunately, this is changing.

Choosing a Doctor

Imagine a foot race over the four hundred meter hurdles. That's once around a track, jumping over barriers all the way around. It is one of the most exhausting and demanding of races. It takes skill, training and endurance. But imagine eight men or women all lined up in a row in the finals of the Olympic games. The gun goes off. They all clear the first hurdle together. At the second, the same. The third they all clear together. This continues all the way around the track. At the finish line, all the athletes cross the line at exactly the same time.

What are the odds of that happening? One million to one? Ten million to one? One billion to one? It's an absurd scenario, because obviously all runners are not equal. Yet the American Medical Association has been accused of that kind of thinking—not admitting there are differences in the ability of physicians and surgeons. The American public knows that not all doctors are equal in ability and training and expertise, but it's awkward when a physician admits there is a difference in ability.

Just How Good Is the Doctor?

So how do you judge physicians and surgeons? Well, it isn't easy. Even doctors frequently aren't good judges. I am frequently amazed by the doctors that doctors seek out for care.

But there are ways to find out. Here are some key questions to ask. Are the physicians "board eligible" or "board certified"? Their office should know the answer. If they hem and haw, then they are not. Board eligibility means that they've completed training and have not yet taken the test because they haven't been in practice long enough or else haven't passed it. Board certified means they have not only completed the training but have passed an exam, a rigorous examination that certifies when they took the exam they were knowledgeable in the area of certification in their specialty. Office staffs will usually answer these questions very willingly if there is nothing to hide.

If you know any nurses or doctors, ask them about a particular doctor. Try and read between the lines with what they say. But usually, you'll get a straight answer if the person you are asking is a friend.

What's His Experience?

If you are seeing a doctor, don't be afraid to ask him what experience he has in treating your condition. If it's surgery, ask him how many of these operations he has done. Obviously, the more experience the doctor has had in treating your problem, the better chance that he is good at it and you are going to have a successful treatment.

Then ask yourself how you feel about the doctor. Can you relate to him? Can you communicate with him? It is important you be convinced you're getting an honest answer and you're not getting the runaround.

Is Being a Christian Important?

Many Christians feel it is important to be treated by a Christian physician. But just because a physician is a Christian does not make him a better physician. I know Christian physicians who are superb physicians or surgeons. I know Christian physicians whose behavior is an embarrassment and bedside manner dismal, but who are technically good. And I know Christian physicians who aren't very good at all. My own recommendation is to make your decision on objective grounds of communication skills and technical ability rather than on beliefs.

Is Bedside Manner Important?

Bedside manner used to be the way physicians were judged. In fact, the classic doctor portrait of the concerned doctor leaning over the bed holding the hand of the sick child is what most people think of when they think of bedside manner. That picture has gone by the wayside as medicine has changed. Nowadays, most physicians have a poor bedside manner or no bedside manner at all!

Is bedside manner important? The answer is yes and no. If you have a problem that requires repeated visits of the doctor over a long period of time, your doctor must understand your situation and needs and goals. Then bedside manner is important. Bedside manner is a healing art. Physicians with good bedside manner tend to touch and hold and are good listeners.

But if your problem is straightforward and technical, for example a difficult surgical challenge that requires highly technical skills, then bedside manner may not be important. What may be important is to see the best surgeon that you can.

Fifty years ago, a doctor faced with a problem they couldn't treat only needed to exercise the healing gifts of touch and listening and compassion and understanding. But as medicine and surgery have become more high tech, bedside manner began to be ignored. Physical touching began to be ignored. The more high tech medicine has become, the less touching it has included and the worse bedside manner has become. Many physicians have found themselves going from the role of healer to the role of technician.

The Three "A's" of Medical Practice

Whenever I'm talking to young doctors, or older ones for that matter, about success in practice, I am reminded of what a professor told me about how to be successful in a medical practice. He said there are three A's that are important. The first A is availability. If you are sick or hurting, and there is only one doctor available, you're going to see that doctor, no matter what you think of him. The one way to be successful is to be available, and that's the most important aspect of "building a successful practice."

The second important A is affability. The better his bedside manner, the friendlier he is, the better communicator he is, the more likely a doctor is to be successful. And in fact, availability and affability are far and away the two most important aspects of being a successful physician or surgeon. If a doctor is available, friendly and communicative, he is going to be successful, unless he's just awful. Most of us judge our doctors on those two A's. Can we get into see them, and are they friendly?

The third A, the least important A in being a successful doctor, is ability. That is also the hardest one to judge.

How to Talk to Your Doctor

Everybody going to see a doctor has questions they want to ask. Being in a doctor's office is highly stressful, and many people forget what they wanted to ask. Write down your questions before you get into the office, or take a friend along with you to remind you and to help you remember the answers. Don't hesitate to take notes. It is amazing to me how little people remember of what they're told.

Here are five key questions to ask about almost any treatment or surgery.

1. What happens if there is no treatment?

Every fall several people come in complaining of popping and grinding in their knees. They have no pain and no disability, but they are worried that they are becoming arthritic because of the noise they've noticed. My advice to them is don't worry about it. As long as it doesn't hurt and you can do the things you want to do, ignore the noise. They leave the office happily and go skiing and are never seen again.

There are many symptoms and conditions that don't need to be treated at all. So ask, "Do I need to treat this symptom or this condition?"

2. What happens if the treatment is successful?

Don had developed an arthritic hip. It became so painful, he could no longer run. He could walk comfortably, he could bicycle, and he could swim, but he was an avid runner. He had seen a orthopedic surgeon who recommended an artificial hip joint for him. I concurred with this opinion; an artificial hip would, if the surgery was successful, significantly relieve his pain. After surgery, he would be forbidden from running because the artificial hip would not stand the rigors of long distance running. Since that was the only time he had his pain, Don decided to hold off on his surgery.

3. What are the chances of success of the treatment, whether it's medical or surgical?

Joyce had a grinding in her knee with minimal discomfort. She could play tennis, bicycle, and walk without difficulty, but she really didn't like the grinding. Her surgeon diagnosed damaged cartilage on her kneecap, and she underwent successful arthoscopic surgery (microscopic removal of the damaged cartilage) in an outpatient operation. The surgeon felt very good about his "successful" surgery because he had removed all the damaged cartilage. But her knee ground even worse than before, and now she was having more pain and was unable to play tennis.

Joyce was very unhappy. She had forgotten to ask what the chances were of relieving the grinding. Her surgeon had misunderstood or wrongly estimated the amount of pain she was having. She misunderstood or forgot what he said about the grinding. Grinding from cartilage on the underside of the knee is hardly ever relieved by surgery on the cartilage. In fact, the noises frequently are worse after surgery. But if there is pain, many times the pain can be successfully relieved. Conversely, if you operate on a painless knee, it can frequently become painful.

Joyce had not asked a critical question. Her surgeon had not communicated to her well. He couldn't understand why she was unhappy with his technically successful surgery.

4. What are potential complications, and what are the chances of their occurring?

There are two parts to this question. All of life is a risk, and many medical treatments are safer than an automobile drive into the city. But medicine is an imperfect science (maybe that's why we "practice" medicine rather than "do" medicine).

Mark had become extremely disabled with back pain. The x-rays showed a very unusual shift in the spine, a reverse shift, which is exceedingly rare. He saw some of the best surgeons in the world and all of them recommended the same procedure—an anterior spinal fusion.

Without the surgery, Mark would live with stiffness and pain. He would no longer be able to play tennis. He would no longer be able to practice his career as a surgeon. But if he had the operation, there was a one to two percent risk that he'd be impotent afterward. Unwilling to take that risk, Mark has accepted the disability.

That's an example of knowing the chance of complications and making a rational decision whether or not you want to take those risks. Some of us may be more willing to accept certain risks than others, and that's fine.

But some complications are unpredictable; why they happen defies earthly explanation. This was the case with Loraine.

A Risk of Complications

Loraine spent a lifetime being a nurse. She was head nurse in a children's rehabilitation hospital and went on to become a specialized enterostomal therapist so she could better care for her osteomy patients. When she retired from the children's hospital, she worked with adults, teaching them how to take care of their osteomies, which are external drainage bags or openings from the bowel or bladder for people who have been paralyzed or had rectal surgery.

She was a loving, giving, caring person. When she retired, her husband became disabled. She nursed and cared for him until he died. Then she was free to do in retirement what she planned. Independent and self-sufficient to a fault, she traveled and visited her grandchildren and enjoyed them immensely. Something Loraine never wanted to do was become dependent upon anyone or require long-term supportive care when there was no hope for recovery. She signed a living will to preclude any heroic measures should she become desperately ill.

One day Loraine noticed a lump in her breast. It got larger and larger. It finally got to the size where she could no longer ignore it. She consulted her family practitioner, who recommended biopsy and surgery. She finally told her daughter; then she again delayed surgery for several months. Finally she had the surgery; it was breast cancer. She had a modified simple mastectomy and only a few lymph nodes were involved. She sailed through the surgery without any difficulty. Her church, her children's churches, and grandchildren's school had prayed for her. However, because of the "aggressive nature" of the cancer, the pathologist, surgeon and family doctor felt that short courses of radiation therapy were appropriate.

Loraine underwent the radiation therapy. Halfway through the treatment she became ill and developed pain in her arm. As the treatments were continued, she lost strength and developed severe disabling pain in her arm requiring injectable pain medication. She grew weak, and her daughter took her into her house. She was no longer independent, but required almost full-time nursing care. With the aid of many nurses and her daughter and grandchildren, she was able to be cared for at home, but it was a struggle.

Then Loraine had a stroke and was taken to the hospital. No heroic measures were performed. She recovered, weakened, and returned to her daughter's home. When her granddaughter was with her, she had a seizure, probably another stroke. Again she was hospitalized. Eventually she was transferred to a rehabilitation hospital, but she was severely handicapped and wheelchair bound. Caring for her became more difficult, but her daughter continued to do so.

Loraine, being fiercely independent and "not wanting to be a burden," fought with her daughter and demanded that she be placed in a nursing home. For the first six months there, she would constantly plead for her daughter to give her enough medication to kill her. She had another stroke, and now she's trapped in a slowly aging and failing body, unable to communicate well.

Loraine had tremendous complications from her radiation therapy, which is really quite rare. Her family practitioner had been in practice for fifty years and had never seen it, nor had her surgeon ever seen it to such a degree. Loraine is a classic example of how things can go wrong in medicine, even when the appropriate things are done. She now finds herself trapped in the one position that she never wanted to be in.

5. How soon must the treatment begin?

In certain life threatening emergencies, there is no doubt that the treatment must be done immediately. In other conditions, a few days or a few weeks won't affect the outcome either way. And there are some conditions that are completely elective, that is, you can have them treated whenever it is a convenient time for you.

There are certain ligament injuries where my advice to the patient differs depending on how long it's been since the time they injured the knee. If I see them within the first week and I suspect a serious injury, we may suggest surgery be done within the first week or ten days from injury. If, however, the patient has procrastinated in coming in, and it has been two weeks since injury for the identical condition, I will then suggest that they not do anything and wait and see how they do. This is because after ten to fourteen days following the injury, shriveling and atrophy has developed so that repair is impossible and reconstruction is necessary. And reconstruction can be done at any time and is much more elective than repair.

The important thing when surgery or treatment is recommended is to ask the doctor how soon you have to start the treatment before there is any harm from delay.

Marjorie came in complaining of knee pain. Her knees ground, made noise, and hurt her when she was very active, but that did not stop her from doing what she wanted to do. I told her what her options were. Number one was simply to put up with the pain and "do her thing." If the pain ever became severe enough, then surgery could be performed. In my opinion, there was no harm in delay of surgery until it was a convenient time for her or until her disability justified it.

Marjorie was relieved and ecstatic when I told her this. She had hidden the fact that she was seeing me as a second opinion. Her first opinion had recommended surgery for the grinding and popping in her knee, and she assumed that the surgery had to be done immediately. It's been two years now and Marjorie still hasn't had her surgery. Her knees still hurt her some, but she is still "doing her thing."

Getting a Second Opinion

When should you get a second opinion? The easiest answer to that is "whenever you think you need one." My own practice on second opinions is that if you completely trust your doctor, if his or her advice makes sense to you, and if he has experience in treating this condition, then a second opinion could be a waste of time and may even add confusion.

But Sometimes—

But sometimes, you really do need a second opinion. Joan came in very agitated and apprehensive. She had very small bunions on her feet. They didn't bother her, they didn't look bad, and she was able to wear shoes without difficulty. I didn't see anything to worry about, so I asked her what the problem was. Joan had been to a health fair and had seen a foot specialist. He told her her bunions were terrible and that she needed major surgery on both bunions or she was going to end up with crippled feet for the rest of her life.

Joan needed the second opinion!

Insurance Requirements

Tim was sixteen. He had an ankle problem and had been treated correctly for two years, but hadn't responded to treatments. Now his surgeon had recommended surgery. The family agreed, Tim agreed, and they wanted the surgeon to do it. Their insurance demanded a second opinion. They saw another orthopedic surgeon who agreed with the diagnosis, but colored and phrased his opinion in such a way as to cast doubt upon the previous treatment and the recommended surgery at this point and time.

I saw them as a third opinion, to break the tie, if you will. They were confused and distraught, concerned that they had not been treated appropriately by the man they had known and trusted for years. I knew the personalities involved with the physicians. I knew that the second opinion giver was jealous of the first, and I felt that he had been unfair in sowing these seeds of distrust.

I fully concurred with the first opinion and told the family this. I also commended the first surgeon on his good job of conservative treatment. Even though it hadn't been successful, I thought it had been textbook and appropriate and told them that. They were very relieved and happy, but had been put through anguish that they didn't need by their insurance company's demands to get a second opinion.

Uncovering the Missed Fact

Joel underwent successful knee surgery after a serious skiing accident. The day of the surgery he was doing fine, but then he got sick. He wasn't running a fever, but he just wasn't doing well. He didn't have an infection, and he hadn't had any other major complications that could be determined. A second opinion from a medical specialist revealed that Joel had become diabetic. He had a strong family history of diabetes and had been tested for diabetes before surgery. But up until now, all the tests had been negative. But now it was clear he had become diabetic and needed intense diabetic treatments. He responded quickly, made an uneventful recovery from his knee surgery, and is successfully treating his diabetes by diet alone.

Second Opinion Guidelines

Deep down, most people know if their doctor is telling them the truth. If they have any question about his advice, or any trouble trusting him, then they need a second opinion.

A second opinion can be helpful when treatment is not going the way you expected or when an extremely difficult problem means two or three heads are better than one. Good physicians or surgeons don't fear second opinions and don't get upset when they're requested. In fact, good physicians and surgeons will sometimes suggest second opinions just to verify that their opinion is correct or to have someone take a fresh look at it. Sometimes, second opinions can be very helpful.

Using the Strengths and Compensating For the Weaknesses of Traditional Medicine

Whereas modern traditional medicine has become poorer at treating certain conditions and poorer in its treatment of people, it also has become technically better in stamping out certain diseases. We are better than ever at treating certain athletic injuries and restoring people to a competitive level sooner than before. We are better able to treat many injuries. We've never been more successful in treating cancers, never been better at treating infections, and we've never been better at prolonging life at both ends of the spectrum from little preemies to the elderly.

Still, ultimate effectiveness of any medical treatment requires a union of patient and procedure. For you to get the most benefit out of traditional medicine, follow these principles.

A. Have Faith in the Treatment
For medicine to be effective, you must have faith that

it is going to be. If you don't believe in the treatment, then you significantly decrease the chances of it being successful. Faith in the treatment is still the key element in success. We will discuss this in greater detail in Chapter 7.

I don't know a surgeon who would operate on a patient who told them, "Doc, I don't believe that I'm going to survive this operation. I really believe I'm going to die under the knife." I personally have canceled surgery in those circumstances and know many other surgeons who feel the same way. To get the most out of medical traditional medicine, you must have faith that it is effective and that God will use it.

B. Get to the Causes

As modern medicine has tended to become more high tech and low touch, doctors have technically become better able to treat people. But modern medicine has seemingly become less well adapted at treating certain entities, such as stress related illness. It can treat the symptoms and signs of the illness: ulcers, migraine, high blood pressure, upper back pain, "fibrositis," eczema, colitis.

Many of these disease processes are caused by stress and then lead to physical ailments. Medicine can be good at defeating the physical ailments, but it is woefully inadequate in helping the person deal with the stress and the root cause rather than the manifestations and the symptoms of the disease. So the problems keep recurring because the cause has not been addressed.

C. Be Motivated to Get Better

There are certain nerve injury conditions which lead to constant or recurring bouts of pain. Once a malady or painful condition has been present or painful for several years' time, the pain is virtually incurable. Patients with chronic pain develop or endure psychological changes as a result of the pain. They become depressed, self-centered, and irritable; their family life and work life are ruined.

Pain centers have a fifty percent success rate; they are very successful in treating chronic pain if they are able to motivate the patient. Success doesn't mean pain relief, but means having the patient functioning back in society in spite of that pain.

D. Remember Christian Principles

Modern medicine is often very poor at handling death and dying. Like all of our society, medicine is goal oriented and success oriented. In medicine, death is the ultimate failure. Medicine has become high tech, but the treatment of dying is low tech, high touch, high caring. The reason the hospice movement has been so successful and grown so rapidly is to fill the void created by modern medicine's inability to deal with death and dying.

Nowhere does one's faith impact as greatly as when faced with an inevitably fatal illness; all normally successful and traditional treatments have failed. This is where having an understanding compassionate physician is all important. An atheistic physician, or a physician of another religion, may not ever be willing to "quit." You have every right to re-ask the questions that we talked about earlier in any part of your treatment. What happens if no treatment is given? What happens if this new treatment that you are recommending is successful? What are the chances of prolonging life or the quality of life? What are the chances of success in this treatment? Is it one percent or ninety percent, or something in between? What are the potential complications and side effects and chances of these complications and side effects? Is this treatment aimed at prolonging life for days or weeks going to make me sick and miserable? Will it do permanent damage to my heart or lungs or brain? How soon must this treatment begin?

Remember that if your physician believes, as pagan America does, that you only go around once and you've got to reach for all the gusto you can this one time, he or she is not going to quit. They will do everything they can to squeeze every hour and minute of life out of your body because, for them, quantity or length of life may be more important than quality. And if in fact you only do go around once, then length of life, regardless of what it's like, may be more important.

E. Consider Other Treatment

A friend called and pleaded with me to see his pastor's wife, "even though she wasn't an athlete." Joanna was having recurring bouts of upper back pain and, it turns out, had seen three doctors already. When I saw her, she was actually quite comfortable.

She was the assistant pastor's wife and had an outside job as a legal secretary. Both of these positions are physically and emotionally stressful. She admitted that she was having difficulty handling the stress, but no one had ever told her that the upper back pain in the back of her lower neck was related to stress. She was quite concerned that it was something far more serious than that. I was able to reassure her that that was not the case, but that the painful bouts were going to continue to recur until she was able to manage her stress. I suggested that she see a local Christian psychologist who counsels in stress management and has demonstrated how prayer and devotions are effective in stress reduction where modern medicine has failed.

The Man Who Couldn't Walk

"Doctor Dominguez, please come to the emergency room. We have a man here who was run over by a car and can't move his leg. But you don't need to sprint down."

When I arrived at the emergency room, there was George on a cart, looking quite comfortable and content. He claimed that he had been hit by a car that tried to run him over! George was a union organizer, and his union was trying to organize a large factory nearby. This is in conservative, Republican DuPage county—not a hot bed of unionism, to say the least.

There were no bruises or bumps on George's body. The x-rays of his spine, his pelvis, and his legs were all normal. His reflexes were all normal. He claimed he had decreased sensation, but could feel a pin everywhere in his legs and felt function returning. There was no objective evidence that George had been seriously injured, yet he claimed he couldn't walk or move his legs. I was dubious.

Nevertheless, we had to admit George for observation. A day later, after one day of physical therapy, George was up walking. After two days of therapy, I told George I thought he would probably be able to go home in the morning. George was very suspicious of this and demanded a second opinion. Later on that morning, I got a frantic call from the nurse that George had collapsed in the bathroom and couldn't move his leg.

George had rung a bell and was found in a heap on the bathroom floor, but no one had seen it happen. He was able to help get himself into bed and didn't have to be carried. I arranged a consultation with a neurosurgeon, a neurologist, and an internal medicine specialist. All four of us came to the same conclusion. George had no objective evidence of paralysis. George had a hysterical conversion reaction. We all agreed on a plan of treatment.

The following morning I presented George with our conclusions and told him that the "good news" was there was no evidence of paralysis. I told him there was some stress and psychological reaction to an incident that happened in the picket lines. It turned out that George was convinced he would be run over if he went back to leading and organizing the strike, which he would have to do if we sent him home. I told George that the only way I could justify keeping him in the hospital was to arrange psychiatric consultation and psychological testing.

George was incensed, called me incompetent, and told me that he was going to find some doctors who could find out what was wrong with him. I told him he would have to see the psychologist the following day or else go home, but I would give him twenty-four hours to think it over before I wrote all of this in his chart.

The nurse called me back later that morning and related that George had again collapsed in the bathroom, claiming his legs had gone out on him. He claimed he was totally paralyzed, although he helped get himself back into the bed. He said he was surrounded by incompetence, then signed himself out of the hospital against medical advice and arranged an ambulance to transfer him to a hospital in Chicago.

It's almost impossible to treat hysterical conversion reaction, because the patients find the consequences of getting better worse than the consequences of being sick. To prove they are right, they have to remain sick. Even with psychology or psychotherapy, the patient has to be better off healthy than sick for them to get better. Until that situation exists, people with a conversion reaction remain "sick."

F. Change Your Lifestyle

Tony's dad died of a stroke when he was forty-seven. Tony, who looked the picture of health, was now twenty-five and had very high blood pressure. He had occasional headaches and dizzy spells. Tony was a fitness buff with a magnificant body. He lifted all the time and worked out very strenuously. His eating habits were erratic. He liked junk food and highly salted foods.

We sent Tony to one of the best internists in town, who evaluated him and had him on a wide variety of medications, all of which had a variety of obnoxious side affects. But Tony never changed his lifestyle or his eating habits, and continued to really push himself in power lifting. He continued to have the symptoms of high blood pressure and the complications of the medications. Eventually he was sent to a prestigious medical center out of town. They did a complete evaluation on him and basically made the same recommendations that the first internist had made. Tony's blood pressure is out of control. True, his family history of high blood pressure plays a significant role in it, but so do his lifestyle and psychological makeup. Even though intellectually and theoretically Tony knows all this, he cannot see the errors in his own lifestyle as causes for his high blood pressure.

Traditional medicine has much to offer, but remember to keep these guidelines in mind as you seek it out.

Choose your doctor as carefully as you can, know how to talk to him, know when to seek out that second opinion, and remember what medicine can and cannot do.

7

The Role of Faith in Medicine

Modern science may have a reputation for being interested only in the cold, clinical, provable-in-the-laboratory facts, but medical personnel are well aware of the role faith plays in the healing process. How else to explain the legendary "placebo effect" or the success stories of groups like Alcoholics Anonymous? In this chapter, we will look closely at some of the ways our faith in the process itself enters into our healing.

Faith in the Treatment

When I was a resident, it was not uncommon for a nurse to come to me and say, "Mr. Jones in Room 303 is taking too much pain medicine, and I don't believe he is hurting. Can't we give him a placebo to prove he's not having pain?"

I would give permission for the injection of an innocuous substance, which the nurse would tell the patient was pain medication. Most of the time, the "ineffective medication" would relieve the pain.

"See!" the nurse would exclaim. "I told you he wasn't hurting in the first place!"

But the truth is that anything that is done to a person

who is in pain, if he is told that what is being done or given to him is effective in relieving pain, will effectively relieve the pain at least fifty percent of the time. Placebos work!

To increase the placebo effect, one need only be more convincing to the sufferer about the effectiveness of the medication. The more trust and faith the patient has in the person who is administering the drug, the stronger and more effective the placebo will be.

The placebo effect is not imaginary. Medical science realizes its effectiveness. However, because it lacks objectivity and smacks of deception, modern medicine makes little use of placebos. In fact, since my first year or so in practice, I have refused to prescribe placebos.

King County Specials

When I was an intern in Seattle at the King County Hospital, all the medications in the outpatient clinic for eligible patients were free. So the medications they stocked were only the basic effective medications. Expensive new pain-relieving drugs were never stocked, but the patients had access to aspirin or codeine if their physicians would prescribe it.

The most popular and most effective oral pain medicine was the "King County pain pills"—acetylsalicylic acid, or aspirin. It's the only place in the country I have seen pink aspirin! Although it was forbidden to use the word aspirin around the patient, one could use the term "acetylsalacidic acid."

Of course, aspirin is a very effective pain reliever, and it is one of the true wonder drugs of our modern age. If you combine an effective medication with a potent placebo effect, you really have something. In King County, we had something! Patients would drive from miles to come back and get the King County pain pills—the "only thing that worked" for them!

The Placebo Effect

Most of us have been exposed to an example of how scientists try to eliminate the placebo effect and really study the effectiveness of a medication with the research on the new drug "AZT," an effective palliation for patients suffering with AIDS. In order to eliminate the placebo effect, all of the patients in the study were warned that they might be receiving a useless substance. Only half of them would be given a medication. Had the patients all been told they were going to receive an effective medication, even in a devastating, fatal illness such as AIDS, scientists knew that improvement and well being, as proven in longevity or in any parameter measure, could simply have been the result of a placebo effect rather than the effectiveness of the drug. Some think this is a cruel form of test, but in fact, it is the only way one can objectively test the effectiveness of a medication.

Rallying the Immune System

Recent research has shown that the mechanism by which faith in your treatment helps bring about healing is by stimulating your immune system to fight disease. The immune system is that in our body which helps us fight off infection and disease. Not only does the immune system help us fight off viruses and bacterial infection, it is one of the important aspects in fighting off cancer and other illnesses as well.

Cancer cells are basically normal cells that have slightly gone wrong and start to grow wildly. Normally the body will recognize these abnormal cells and destroy them before they can get too big and overpower the body's immune system. Most of us frequently have cancer cells floating around in our bodies, but they are killed because the body recognizes them as abnormal. Our immune system is what keeps us free from disease.

The reason AIDS is such a deadly disease is that it is the first disease process known to directly attack the immune system. What kills in AIDS is not the AIDS virus, but the lack of immunity caused by the AIDS virus. It kills our immune system and then our bodies are defenseless to fight off a host of otherwise relatively innocuous infections.

The Effectiveness of "Right Thinking"

Another way that faith and meditation help with healing is by seeing ourselves getting better or seeing an infection beaten back or seeing a tumor shrink. We can't directly control lower body function, that is our heart rate, circulation to our hands and feet, skin temperature, circulation to organs. That is controlled by a "lower" part of the brain that is not under direct voluntary control. But through biofeedback it is possible for people to learn how to control these functions.

When we say run faster, our muscles help us run faster. The lower part of our brain doesn't react to commands the way we normally do; rather, it relies on visual images. We can't simply teach ourselves to relax muscles, but if we can visualize ourselves lying on a raft floating in a swimming pool with the warm sun beating down on us, we can communicate that to our lower brain and hence to our involuntary nervous system, and thereby exercise control over these lower functions.

Cancer therapists make use of biofeedback training by telling patients, "When I give you this medication, I want you to 'see it' going to the tumor and killing it." Or, "When we give you this radiation, we want you to see the radiation killing the tumor cells—killing just the tumor and nothing else." They have discovered that visualizing treatments at work is an effective way of improving the success rate of their cancer treatments.

Psychologists have long known that the pain in the upper back can be relieved by relaxing the muscles through biofeedback training. It can also be used to reduce blood pressure.

The fact that there are psychological and physiological explanations for how faith helps in the healing process in no way diminishes its role. God uses your belief that your treatment is going to work to rally your body's defense system and help you recover.

Faith in the "Treater"

Faith in the medication or treatment being given is one important component of healing. Another is confidence in the person administering the treatment.

Tom was a jock who lived to play sports. He worked hard and he played hard and then he injured his knee. It repeatedly locked on him. To his chagrin he realized that in trying to save a few bucks on insurance, he had signed up with an HMO. Now he had to see a family doctor he didn't know rather than a sports medicine specialist.

He grudgingly went to see the family doctor, who told him the x-rays in his exam were okay and not to worry. He continued to have trouble and went back several times and demanded to see an orthopedic surgeon, a sports medicine specialist. His HMO doctor sent him to see an orthopedic surgeon whom he didn't get along with and he was told he had a torn cartilage. Surgery was recommended.

I saw him in consultation and concurred with the diagnosis. He expressed frustration that I couldn't do his surgery because of the insurance plan he was in. He had to have this other physician do the surgery or pay for all his hospital charges and my fee out of his own pocket. The other way it would cost him nothing. I suggested he go ahead and have the other surgeon do it, since I knew he was a capable surgeon.

Tom didn't want to do it. He didn't trust or like the other doctor, but nevertheless he went through with the surgery. Two weeks later he was not fully recovered and having some pain. The physician gave him some exercises and told him not to do sports for three months.

I saw Tom back in consultation two days later. He was upset and agitated. When I examined him, he looked terrific. He still had some weakness that would respond to therapy and exercise, and I told him this. I told him his knee was fine, and he could go back to sports in just a few weeks if he did what his other physician had told him. He was elated and asked if he could see me one more time in a month. When I saw him, he was ecstatically playing sports and feeling fine.

The point is, even a routine, minor operation that shouldn't require much faith at all does require faith. Until you have faith in what your physician or surgeon is telling you and in his ability to treat you, his treatment isn't going to work.

Faith in God

The atheist head of an internationally famous drug rehabilitation program in southern California said that in all his years of working with substance abuse and alcoholism, he has never seen anyone cured of addiction to hard drugs who has not had a significant life-changing religious experience.

In addition to faith in the treatment and faith in the person providing the treatment, there is a third important ingredient for healing, which Christians have recognized all along: faith in God. A non-Christian scientist or secular organization, like Alcoholics Anonymous, might express it as faith in a "higher power."

Alcoholics Anonymous' credo and its plan for successfully treating and managing alcohol requires that the alcoholic admit their failure to handle their problem. They must admit they are alcoholic. And they must admit deep down inside they'll always be an alcoholic. They must admit they need help outside of themselves to conquer alcoholism. They are going to have to rely on this outside power as well as their fellow converted alcoholics in AA for support and to help keep them dry. Furthermore, AA meetings are punctuated by testimonials and confessions of alcoholics.

Then there's Weight Watchers, a kind of modified "foodaholics anonymous." They too rely on open meeting testimonials and confessions about how much they weigh, how much they want to lose, their successes and failures of the past week in combating the demon food.

Starting With "Confession"

There are many medically effective cures for various substance abuse problems. That is not to say they are valueless; the opposite is true. It is interesting to compare the techniques used in these programs. Basically they are aimed at educating and convincing the person that they have a problem, that they are in fact substance abusers. First, the patients must come to a conclusion that they have a problem. Once they have "confessed" to this problem, then they start to work through the problem and try to start over again. Without help outside of themselves, they are not going to make it.

The similarities between these public meetings and old fashioned revival meetings is striking. But instead of confessing sin and asking for God's forgiveness and help, people are confessing to a need for alcohol or food and the ability to control that.

The Life-Changing Experience

But the one true life-changing, person-changing, habit-changing religious experience is being born again. Every evangelical church has members of its congregation for whom this life-changing religious experience has also been the path to salvation from alcohol, drug abuse, addiction to gambling, wife beating, etc.

Being born again, having a relationship with Jesus Christ, is the ultimate life-changing experience and is the number one way that God heals. Having confessed that we are sinners and that there is nothing that we can do about it, we accept God's freely given forgiveness and are born again into God's family. This is a dramatic, life-changing experience.

For the substance abuser, it is the one effective cure-all. While some say that their craving for alcohol or cocaine or cigarettes never goes away, there are many who testify that the craving itself is removed.

Being born again is the one authentic spiritual experience with an everlasting cure. Other "spiritual experiences" can help, but they're not the real thing. There is no substitute for salvation. And when it is all said and done, it is the effective treatment for substance abuse.

Living in an Imperfect World

While being born again is the ultimate life-changing experience, the problem we face in our society is that many people use it as a cop-out and a solution to all the problems of the world. They think that all of their problems will go away. They think that all of their unhealthy desires and cravings will instantly go away. They will instantly become successful, happy, fulfilled, with no family problems, job problems, financial risks, stresses, or anxieties.

Of course, this isn't the case. We still live in an imperfect world. We are all imperfect sinners. Accepting Jesus Christ doesn't mean that you will be transported instantly to a perfect world, to live in perfectly blissful surroundings.

The most common way a born again person is healed is by an ever growing desire to please God and follow his mission—including his good health guidelines that we outlined in Chapter 5. Once you are a child of God, you are going to do what your Father wants. You want to please your Father, and wanting to please Him makes Him want to bless you.

Seeing the Physician

Remember that there are no Biblical references that say one ought *not* to seek a physician. In Matthew 9:12, Jesus said, "It is not the healthy who need a doctor, but the sick." The implication is that it is logical to see a doctor when you are sick.

Stories from both Old and New Testaments reinforce this. "In the thirty-ninth year of his reign, Asa was afflicted with a disease in his feet. Though his disease was severe, even in his illness he did not seek help from the

Lord, but only from physicians—in the forty-first year of his reign Asa died" (II Chronicles 16:12-13). It was not for going to doctors that Asa was judged, but for not seeking God's intervention *as well*.

"Then Isaiah said, 'Prepare a poultice of figs.' They did so and applied it to the boil, and he recovered"(II Kings 20:7). Certainly Isaiah could have prayed for healing without applying a poultice, but the treatment was recommended, and recovery occurred.

"She has suffered a great deal under the care of many doctors and had spent all she had, yet instead of getting better she grew worse" (Mark 5:26). Jesus did not criticize the woman for seeking physicians, but in her extremity he healed her completely and permanently.

In all of these examples, the implication is that the treatments and medicine were reasonable and right.

Today's "Miracle Drugs"

As we noted in Chapter 2, many of the ailments and diseases treated miraculously by Christ and the apostles now can be treated by modern medicine and surgery—dropsy, dysentery, fever, infection, cataracts, leprosy, seizures, and female bleeding, to name just some. There are "miracle drugs" available now and "miracles" of modern surgery that were not even imagined in the first century.

I believe that God uses miraculous healing much more in third world countries, divorced from the benefits of modern medicine, than He does in our society.

In all this I do not mean to imply that modern medicine and surgery have now supplanted or are now possessors of the "gift of healing." I think they are not. But more often than not, God uses our faith in the "mud, spit, and fingers" of Western medicine, as discussed in this chapter, to bring about our healing. This does not detract from the quality of the healing, nor deny that it ultimately comes from God. You are no less healed if you have been healed by the miracle of surgery or by a miracle drug than if you are healed by a touch.

8

What About "Real" Healing?

So God works through modern medicine, and through our own bodies, to bring us back to health. But what about "real" healing—the instantaneous, unexplainable, supernatural kind, like that performed by Christ and the apostles in New Testament times?

All believers agree that God still *can* do miraculous healing; to deny that is to deny that our God is omnipotent. At Lourdes there is a wall of names of people who have been healed there, miraculously. But the debate comes over how often God does this, and whether or not we can *expect* Him to do it whenever we ask. Those names on the wall at Lourdes are only a few of the hundreds of thousands of people who visit that place each year, hoping to be healed.

Is Any One of You Sick?

"Is any one of you sick? He should call the elders of the church to pray over him and anoint him with oil in the name of the Lord. And the prayer offered in faith will make the sick person well; the Lord will raise him up. If he has sinned, he will be forgiven. Therefore confess your sins to each other and pray for each other so that you may be healed. The prayer of a righteous man is powerful and effective" (James 5:14-16).

Some people believe that everyone who follows this Scripture and has faith will be healed of illness! On the other hand, there are churches where the elders refuse even to do this scriptural injunction. So how do we determine the true Christian perspective on healing? Let's take a closer look at what this passage says.

Call the Elders

First of all, it's interesting to note that it says "call the elders of the church together." It does not say, "call someone in the church who has the gift of healing." The implication here is that all of the elders of the church have the gift or ability to pray over someone and heal them. The passage further implies that the gift of healing is widespread and not unusual.

Notice that it does not say hold a congregational meeting or pray in front of the whole church. My mental picture of this gathering is of you and the elders, not you and the entire congregation. That's not to say that it is wrong to have the entire congregation present, but it is not called for in this verse.

Pray and Anoint

Nowhere in the Bible are the sick advised to seek out a "healer," although there are many references to seeking physicians. So if the elders of your church or the deacons (or the mature believers in the church, if your church does not have an organization of elders or deacons), do pray over you and lay their hands on you or even anoint you with oil, and you have faith that God can heal you, and have asked Him to do so, then you have met the Scriptural standard.

If the elders have prayed over you and you're still not

better, then the action of seeking out a healer may say that you don't trust the faith and prayers of your elders. On the other hand, if the elders of your church won't pray over you or lay hands on you, then I think it is appropriate to seek out a group of believers who will.

The Lord Will Raise Him Up

The second thing to notice about this verse is that it does *not* say that the prayer offered in faith will always make the sick person well. Although many people believe that is the implication, the reality is that it does not always happen!

Remember the examples from Scripture of those who were not healed: Timothy, Trophimus, and Paul, to cite a few. And remember the wall of names at Lourdes of those who experienced documented miraculous healings—a small percentage of the hundreds of thousands who visit each year and who, like the lame and sick gathered at the Pool of Siloam, came hoping for physical wholeness.

If you seek out a healer or a special location because you doubt the faith of your local group of believers, then you need to do some real soul searching as to the faith of your fellow parishioners, the theology of your congregation, or your own faith. Many sincere Roman Catholic believers travel to Lourdes with the hope that a miracle will occur, yes, but also with the realistic expectation that they will be blessed. There is a fellowship of suffering and a comaraderie present in a place like Lourdes that is uplifting and beneficial and can lead to a healing of the spirit, even if it does not lead to a miraculous physical healing. I believe that in that spirit, seeking out this type of experience is valuable and beneficial, and can be a blessed experience.

Three Who Were Healed

Having looked at this key passage in James, on which so much of our theology of healing is based, let's hear the stories of three people who did experience supernatural healing.

Christy

Christy was legally blind in one eye. Her vision was 20/200 and her other eye was normal. Her ophthalmologist was a friend who was a returned missionary from China and founder of one of the great eye clinics in the Midwest. He had treated her for several years. Then she began to lose vision in her good eye. She developed what is called tunnel vision. Tunnel vision is the classical "hysterical conversion reaction" and can be developed between the eye and the brain. Both function normally, but for some psychological reason, the patient loses the ability to see. It's similar to battlefield paralysis—when in the heat of battle or facing battle, a young man became paralyzed and unable to go to war. The eye works, the brain sees what the eye sends it, but then denies it is seeing because of psychological or psychiatric stress.

This young woman was becoming progressively blind in her good eye. The tunnel vision worsened and worsened. Her doctor tried to talk with her and treat her in every way he could, and finally told her that there was nothing else he could do. The problem was psychological. He was going to refer her to a psychologist to help her treat this, because she was legally blind in one eye and becoming functionally blind in the other.

Christy said, "Thank you, doctor, but that's not going to be necessary. I'm going to a healing service next week and I fully expect the Lord to heal me and restore my vision. I will come back in several weeks and check with you."

Christy went to the healing service, claimed to have been healed, and began to see better instantly.

When she returned to have her eyes objectively tested, her vision in the good eye was normal again, the tunnel vision was completely cured, but the bad eye remained 20/200.

Anna Marie

Anna Marie was having repeated bouts of asthma. The wheezing and shortness of breath became progressively worse. She was treated by one of the best doctors in the area and had been to several specialists. She tried various medications and treatments but none of them worked.

Anna Marie asked the elders of her church to pray for her. They prayed over her, laid hands on her at the same time, and she was instantly cured of her statis asthmaticus.

Bronco

Bronco was a retired professional football player. He was a linesman, very good looking, happily married. He was becoming a very successful salesman. He had made the transition from professional football player into the "real world" quite well. As a player he had had back pain on and off, but now his pain became severe. It was a physical battle for him to function daily. He saw several back specialists, chiropractors, and therapists, but nothing helped. His back pain continued to get worse.

He became a born again Christian and began attending a charismatic church. There he noticed the healing that was occurring in the services. He asked the ministers and elders to pray over him. They did, and he was instantly healed of back pain. He has been free of back pain since that time.

Why Christian Physicians Don't Say Much

Most Christian physicians say very little when "faith healing" is discussed in Sunday school. This is a bit unusual, since most physicians I know are opinionated and vocal on most subjects! But when the topic is faith healing, many of us keep our mouths shut rather than appear cynical or squelch the conversation.

Physicians have a strong scientific bias, and acceptance of the scientific method in analyzing illness is taught in medical schools. The scientific method teaches an inherent skeptical prejudice to all phenomena. An even bigger problem for physicians is that many people who claim to have been healed by faith were never physically sick in the first place. Many of the most dramatic requests for "physical healing" are really for emotional illnesses or problems. In watching healing services on television, it is easy to remain skeptical, because one sees little objective evidence of physical illness in most of the "healed."

The three stories told in the previous section are typical of the types of healing that occur at most healing services. All three of these people had failed to respond to standard medical treatments. In fact, all of them were at the end of their ropes because medicine had "done all it could." Their cases were all considered hopeless or incurable. All of them were completely and "miraculously" cured of their symptoms. All of them have remained cured since the time of their healing.

They consider themselves miraculously healed, and they praise God for it.

"Miraculous"

No one, Christian or atheist, would deny that any of these three people were healed. The argument would occur over using the word "miraculous." To the medical scientist or physician, the things about these three cases that stand out are that pain and psychological components are predominant features of these illnesses. Hysterical conversion reaction and status asthmaticus have marked, if not total, psychological components. Pain is impossible to document and measure, so one can never prove the presence or absence of pain. Chronic pain, pain that lasts a long time, has significant psychological factors that come into play because pain changes the psychology of the person.

Secondly, while the symptoms were completely relieved, the physical defects were not completely restored to normal. Bronco's back x-rays looked the same before and after he was healed. The arthritic spurrs that were present before were still present afterwards. The wear and tear that was obvious on x-rays was still obvious on his x-rays. Christy's bad eye was 20/200 before she was healed, and remained 20/200 after she was healed. It was the vision in the good eye that was restored.

When Christ and the apostles healed, diseased tissue was restored to absolute normal appearance and function. Withered tissue, atrophied tissue, was instantly restored to full normal functioning tissue. The scars of leprosy were completely relieved. The person looked cured and was normal.

Christ's Miracles Defied All Physical Law

Skeptical physicians, and even skeptics who aren't physicians, like to point out that many of the successful examples from healing services are from primarily psychologically related illnesses or from painful conditions. To a certain extent this is "sour grapes," because most of these examples aren't well treated or can't be treated at all by modern medical science. Because modern medicine does a poor job, there is a tendency to minimize the importance of such ailments or look discouragingly on the sufferers—and even more discouragingly on successful treatments of the sufferers.

They're not miracles in the same sense that the healings that Christ and the apostles did were miraculous. Christ's miracles defied all physical law, all of the body's natural healing tendencies. He restored dead tissue to health and restored aged and damaged tissue to normal, and nothing in medicine has ever been able to do that.

The healing in hysterical conversion reactions, psychological problems, chronic pain problems, and painful conditions doesn't defy the laws of nature or the concept of normal healing capacity. But just because a physician or medical scientist or skeptic does not consider this "miraculous" does not negate the healing that occurred.

Another point of contention are instances when a cancer or tumor suddenly begins to shrink away, and the body's previously defeated immue system is able to regroup and fight off an illness that had formerly failed to respond to any treatment. Medicine won't call these occurrences miracles; it just throws them into a grab bag of unexplained events known as "spontaneous remission."

Heal with Surgery

Every now and then a person will ask me to heal them with surgery. Like every other surgeon in the world, I have to say that I have no capacity to heal them of anything. I can cut the body open, I can sew it up, I can cut things out, I can plate things back together, I can screw things back together, and I can sew things back up, but that's all I can do. I can't make the incision heal or the blood clot or the scar tissue form.

Physicians can diagnose and dispense medication, and commonly a patient will respond and get better, if the diagnosis is correct and the proper medication given. However, the physician does not heal. All healing ultimately is a gift from God.

Praying for the Surgeon

I've been practicing orthopedic surgery in the "new Jerusalem" of Wheaton, Illinois for over fifteen years now. I routinely pray before every office day and day in the operating room. On those that I haven't, it seems things didn't go as well for me, so I am fearful of missing my prayers before my office hours or surgeries. But in all those years, I can think of only three times when a group has committed to pray for me while I have been in surgery. There may have been more; I certainly hope so. But on three occasions I was told right before surgery that a group was going to pray for me during surgery. All three times the patient was severely injured, the surgery was going to be quite difficult and extensive, and the outcome was unclear.

But these three times stick in my mind because, in spite of the severity of the injury and the difficulty of the surgery, everything went beautifully. I was brilliant! I was better than I knew how to be, and I knew it. Each time I had the sensation that old time evangelists referred to when they spoke of feeling the power of the Spirit.

The surgeries went well, and I knew why. When I talked to the families afterwards and told them how well the surgery had gone, I did credit their prayers. To this day I know they consider me a brilliant surgeon, but I know that even though the surgery was brilliantly done, it was not my brilliance. What I did was beyond my own ability.

The Power of Group Prayer

The fact remains that there is special power in group prayer. The special prayer of Christian healing can make any surgeon brilliant. You have the ability to do that, simply by getting a group of your fellow believers together and making a covenant or pact to pray for that surgeon before and during the surgery. Or pray for the physician or physicians while they are diagnosing and beginning treatment on your friend or loved one. If you want to "test the effectiveness of your prayers," tell that surgeon or physician that you are praying for them and that you are going to pray for their wisdom and their technical ability.

God uses the prayers of elders and the prayers of all of us to aid in healing. It may be through the mud, spit, and fingers of modern medicine, or it may be instant and spectacular. In either case, the healing comes from God.

9

Misunderstanding the Truth

I am thrilled when my patients experience healing. When they are believers, there is a special joy in acknowledging God's healing touch together.

But in my practice, I have dealt with many Christians who, in my opinion, have sadly misunderstood what God's Word has to say about healing, at the cost of considerable pain and anguish to themselves and their loved ones.

In this chapter, we will look at some of these misinterpretations: 1) that we will always be healed, if we have adequate faith, 2) that healing must always mean full restoration, 3) that healing must come by faith alone, without medication or surgery, and 4) that all sickness is a result of sin and can be overcome by "getting right with the Lord."

"We Must Always Be Healed"

Miriam was a lovely Christian girl, the hard-working secretary of one of my best friends. She belonged to a rapidly growing fundamental charismatic church.

"The prayer offered in faith will make the sick person well," James 5:15 says. Miriam and her church firmly believed that whatever your illness or infirmity, God would heal you if you had enough faith.

Miriam's fiance, Jim, also believed as she did. He was drafted and went to Vietnam, where he was shot in the head. He survived the injury, which in itself was a medical miracle. Some physicians might debate whether it was a "good" miracle or one that should not have been performed, but nevertheless he survived. Miriam saw this as God's answer to her prayers to protect her fiance.

After a long hospitalization in the Philippians, and then in an army rehabilitation hospital, Jim was discharged and transferred to the local VA hospital for rehabilitation. He was severely brain damaged. He was quadriplegic, and with supports was able to sit up in a wheelchair. There were times when he would stop breathing and require a respirator.

Before his injury, the wedding day had been set. Miriam refused to alter the plans, for she thought this would demonstrate a lack of faith. Miriam's parents, her fiance's parents, and her church all felt that the wedding should go on as planned; they believed that if she married Jim, he would be healed. The church prayed for him and laid hands on him, and they expected a miracle. My friend was concerned. He asked my opinion, for not only was he losing a very good secretary, but he was concerned for what Miriam's future might hold if she went ahead with her plans.

Given the facts as I heard them, but having never seen Jim, I felt there was little hope for recovery. In fact, I questioned whether the young man had the mental capacity to even legally consent to the wedding. But, since no one on either side of the family was going to contest it, and the minister was willing to perform the ceremony; the wedding was going to proceed.

My concern for Miriam was that not only would her fiance not be healed, but she was committing herself to full-time exhausting nursing care, since she planned to take him out of the hospital and care for him at home—another "demonstration of faith."

I was afraid that the situation would severely tax her faith. I had seen many believers become upset with God, question His judgment, and even reject their faith because of tragic illnesses which failed to respond to prayer. After the wedding, Miriam took Jim home. His condition deteriorated and he had to be rehospitalized. She brought him home again. He deteriorated further and had to be hospitalized again.

My medical opinion proved to be correct. After two and a half years of this repeated scenario, Jim died. Fortunately, I was wrong regarding the spiritual testing. Miriam at no point rejected her faith.

But this is a classic example of how misunderstanding certain passages of Scripture can lead one astray. If we are gung-ho about gifts and need to show off our faith, we are violating the sense of Paul's preaching in II Corinthians and behaving in an unchristian manner. The test of our faith is how we view Christ, not whether or not our faith has the power to heal someone.

Most of us are going to be sick at one time or another in our lives, and all of us are going to die. For some of us that will be sooner than for others.

"We Only Need Faith"

There are at least two books on the market written by parents whose children died because the parents did not seek medical attention. In both instances, the families were encouraged and exhorted by their minister and church (some would say cult) not to seek medical attention. In both these sad instances, the parents had faith that God would heal their children, and in one instance they actually discontinued what had been successful treatment because it seemed to demonstrate a lack of faith.

If we refuse medical or surgical care and treatment, then we will reap the natural history of the disease process. We may get better. We may get worse. We may end up crippled. We may die.

"Having Faith in Faith Alone"

It was late in the evening when I got a call from the emergency room. The physician said, "We have a man here who fell off a ladder and shattered his knee. We can splint it, and you can see him in the morning, but we're sure it's going to require surgery. He's in too much pain to go home."

I said it was no problem, to just splint him and I'd check him in the morning and we could talk about surgery.

"Yes," he said, "there is a problem. He's a Christian Scientist and won't permit any medication or blood transfusion. He doesn't believe in surgery, but he's too disabled to go home."

I said, "Okay, splint him and admit him and don't prescribe any medication."

The next morning I met with Edward, the patient, examined him, and reviewed his x-rays. He had split the upper end of his thigh bone into three pieces. Without major orthopedic surgery with plates and screws, he would probably never walk again.

He was a practicing, believing Christian Scientist. His faith was sorely taxed by his situation. I told him I sympathized with his dilemma, but that I still had to recommend surgery. If he refused, I would try to treat him as best I could, but he would have to realize that the chance of success was minimal. Without surgery, I felt he would never walk again.

He asked if he had a day to think about it, and I said yes. I could see he was suffering and suggested he take pain medicine. He told me he didn't want to take medicine and under no circumstances would he consent to blood transfusions. I was willing to comply with that. I felt that we could probably do the surgery without blood transfusions. If they proved to be necessary, I promised to discuss it with him and let him refuse to take them after he fully understood the consequences.

Some fellow church members met with Edward and some type of doctrinal position was reached. Edward wasn't jeopardizing his faith by consenting to surgery, as long as there were no blood products used and all medication used was related only to the performing of the surgery and anaesthesia. It was easy to stretch this into giving him pain medicine after surgery as part of his post anesthetic recovery.

Edward underwent successful surgery. We did not even need to consider transfusion, and the surgery went well. He took pain medicine for one day, made a remarkable recovery, went on to uneventful healing, and was able to lead a perfectly normal life after that surgery. As far as I know, he is still a practicing Christian Scientist today.

Perhaps you're thinking, "Well, that just shows you how misled those Christian Scientists are. I'm glad I don't believe their doctrine." But there are many fundamental Christians who share this approach to medicine, thinking that since God *can* heal without the "assistance" of medicine, then He must always "prefer" to do it just that way.

Demanding that God heal us without medicine or surgery is putting God to the test. If we fall out of a third story window, it certainly is possible that we may not be hurt or killed. God could use His angels to buoy us up. We could bounce off an awning. The fire department may come by with a rescue net. There may be a swimming pool underneath the window. All of us believe that God could spare us if we fell or jumped out a third story window. But none of us believe that if we did it intentionally as a test that God would protect us. He could, but chances are He won't.

So don't put all your faith in faith alone. Welcome the mud, spit, and fingers of medicine. You are no less healed if you are healed after taking antibiotics or having surgery—the healing still comes from God.

"Getting Off the Medicine"

Ingrid came up to me and said, "Dr. Dominguez, do you know a Christian neurologist in town I can see?" I stated that I wasn't sure what their faith was, but I named all the neurologists in town. She had seen every one of them.

Ingrid had a history of a seizure disorder. Seizures are frequently the result of small areas of scar tissue or abnormalities in the brain that create abnormal electrical stimuli. On medicine for ten years, Ingrid had not had a seizure in that time. She had no side affects from the medicine, had been functioning normally, attended school, and was gainfully employed in an excellent job.

But Ingrid had gone to a healing service where she was told if she had adequate faith, she would be healed. Convinced she had been healed at the service, she went to one of the neurologists I had named, who consented to take her off her seizure medicine to let her "prove" her healing.

Appropriately, he warned her that coming off of seizure medicine too fast could result in seizures or she might not be healed and the seizures could recur if she came off. The man was an excellent neurologist and outlined an appropriate "tapering off" program of her seizure medicine. The minute she was totally off her seizure medicine, she had another grand mal seizure. Her neurologist put her back on her medication.

Ingrid's condition was completely controllable by medication. As a physician, I say that God had already answered her prayer. Yet she was distressed. Convinced that healing had to mean complete restoration and no more medicine, Ingrid was, in my opinion, demanding that the "thorn in her flesh" be removed.

Praying for the Same Anna Marie

Paul prayed three times to have the thorn in his flesh removed. He was told because of his great faith and his relationship with the Holy Spirit, it was not going to be removed for his own good. We can't demand that the thorns in our flesh be removed. They are there for our own spiritual or even physical good. God does not need us to be perfect physical specimens without scars or blemishes to use us to further his kingdom or to bless us.

Contrast Ingrid's story with that of Anna Marie—the same Anna Marie whose miraculous healing from asthma we recounted in Chapter 8. Anna Marie began to suffer severe back pain. She sought physicians and underwent surgery and multiple treatments, but her back pain worsened until it became chronic and disabling.

Every doctor that saw her said there was nothing else they had to offer; she would have to "live with the pain." When the pain was severe, she was virtually immobile. Again Anna Marie sought the elders to pray over her and touch her. She certainly had faith that she could be healed—it had happened to her before.

Her mother sat outside the small room where the elders were praying over Anna Marie, fully expecting her to come bounding out of the room totally cured. The elders prayed, the Spirit of God was present . . . but her pain did not go away. The thorn remained. But Anna Marie still believes there was a healing at that second prayer meeting—a healing of her spirit. She is still physically disabled at times, but she has accepted the pain and has grown spiritually. Even though she did not get the physical healing she had prayed for and fully expected to have, she feels she was spiritually healed.

Just Claiming the Victory

Fred was an accountant in his mid fifties who loved to play tennis. I saw him because he had twisted his knee and whenever he tried to play tennis, the knee would pain him. On my examination he had all the signs and symptoms of a torn knee cartilage.

I told him what I thought he had and felt that in order for him to return playing tennis, he would require arthroscopic surgery of the knee and that, if there were no arthritic changes in the knee, he had a very good chance of being pain free and returning to tennis.

Fred never scheduled a surgery. A year later I saw him again, but this time he was complaining of pain in the other knee. His findings were identical. I gave him the same speech, that I thought that he had a degenerative tear of the cartilage, which is typical of men that age.

He then asked me to check the knee I had diagnosed a year ago. My findings were virtually the same. The same swelling clearly indicated to me that the cartilage had been torn and, in fact, he had a small cyst on his cartilage. He related that he had been pain free now for six months and been able to play tennis, and he wanted me to tell him that the cartilage had healed itself completely and was back to normal. I asked him why.

He said, "Doc, you may not understand this, but I am a charismatic Roman Catholic Christian. I believe in healing and belong to a charismatic group. It's very important for me that I be able to 'claim the victory' of this cartilage being back to normal. Until it's back to normal, I can't 'claim the victory,' and I desperately want to." This was in the midst of a busy office session, and I desperately wanted more time to sit down and talk with him.

I told him that in my view he could "claim the victory" on several accounts. First of all, he had been painless for six months. He had complete relief of his symptoms and was back playing tennis. That in itself was a victory; all I ever hope for in surgery is to relieve the symptoms and restore the person to normal function, not necessarily to normal anatomy. I also had to tell him that his physical examination was exactly the same as it had been a year ago and that I could not change my diagnosis or opinion.

In the short period of time that I had, I tried to reassure him that he did have his victory because the cartilage was no longer bothering him; it didn't matter whether or not it had regenerated itself and healed. At times torn cartilages will get out of the way and quit hurting, especially the degenerative tear. I suggested that if it were to become painful in the future and he did require surgery, in my opinion that would not be defeat, because even then he would still be healed after surgery if it went well and he did not have arthritis in the knee.

I think he clearly understood what I said. I'm not sure whether he accepted it, but he was clearly somewhat relieved by our conversation.

My concern for Fred is twofold. The first is that he still has all the signs, although none of the symptoms, of a torn cartilage in his knee. While he is still playing tennis, he is only playing doubles because his other knee is holding him back from stressing the "healed knee"—the "victorious knee." And while it's not bothering him now, I'm afraid that it will flare up again on him and he may be spiritually defeated by this flare-up.

From a physician's perspective, this is not a serious problem. From a spiritual perspective, it's a major struggle. Degenerative tears of knee cartilages are common in middle aged people. It would be relatively easy and routine to treat Fred in his knee if he were to come to surgery.

My other concern about Fred is his longing to grow spiritually. For Fred, spiritual growth can only be accomplished by full miraculous restoration of a torn degenerative part. Even if he is well and it doesn't hurt, he has to be restored to anatomic normality for the "victory" to be complete.

Don't misunderstand me; miraculous healing can occur. God's healing occurs commonly and frequently, but nowhere in the Bible is restoration to full normal health a step to spiritual growth. In fact, the Bible points out that spiritual maturity comes out of increased testing. "My strength is made perfect in weakness."

While my hope and desire is for all of us is to have victory over illness and injuries, we never should use that victory as a measure of our spirituality. It is not scriptural to claim it. Nowhere does the Bible say we will be restored to normal bodies in this life, that the affects of aging will be banished, or scars be removed.

"Illness is the Result of Sinful Behavior"

In the high school class of one of my children, there was a debate whether illness was a result of sinful behavior. One side argued that all sickness and disability is a direct result of our sinful behavior or God's punishment for sin. It was interesting that the majority of the class seemed to support this position.

Many Christians hold this view. My observation is that those who do have never been seriously ill or injured. Until one has been through that caldron of suffering and pain, it's an easy view to hold.

While there is no question that sickness and disability can be the result of punishment, or the result of volitional choices that we have made, it also can be God's way of blessing us or God doing it for our own good. (These possibilities were discussed in detail in Chapters 3 and 4.) It is clearly a distortion to think that everyone who is sick is being punished for their sin.

Unfortunately, many believers who hold to this opinion will learn that this is not true through their own experience, when they have to face the reality of their own illness or a loved one's suffering. Then they will be forced to rethink their position.

"If You Just Get Right With the Lord..."

When my sister and brother-in-law's baby son was afflicted with cancer, they sought prayer at their church. We prayed at our church for them. All their friends prayed at their churches, but "Ace" did not respond to two traditional surgeries and chemotherapy.

Some people came to their door and told them they were led by the Lord to call on them. If they would pray with them and "get right with the Lord," Ace would be healed. They prayed with these people on several occasions. They strove mightily "to get right with the Lord," but their son continued to deteriorate.

A year and a half later, when I was in Joe Bayly's Sunday school class on death and dying, he related that whenever a Christian is stricken with a severe case or apparently incurable cancer, "false prophets" will show up and tell the affected that they had been led by the Lord to come see them. If they get right with God and pray with them, these people claim, they will be cured. Joe stated categorically that these people were false prophets and their message was spiritually wrong and destructive.

I was thunderstruck, because I had seen this very scenario worked out. I call these false prophets "cancerophiles." There are certain criteria that are always the same when these people show up.

First, it is a believer who is stricken with cancer. Second, the condition has to be serious or apparently near fatal and is not responding to treatment. Third, these cancerophiles do not belong to the sick person's church and in fact are unknown to them. They appear out of the blue. Fourth, their message is always the same—they have been "led by the Lord" and if the sick person or family "gets right with the Lord," they will be healed.

Of course the believer, under great stress because of the illness, welcomes having an apparent fellow believer come over and offer to pray with them. It is natural to seek out prayer when we are ill.

But these people are false prophets. First of all, how do they know you are not "right with the Lord"? No one but God can judge that. Anyone who suggests that you are not right with God is judging you and is sent by Satan to seduce you away with a message that is false.

Don't misunderstand. People you know, fellow members of your church who want to come pray with you, should be encouraged to do so. But these cancerophiles are people unknown to you. If such people show up at your door, do not invite them in. You can thank them for their concern and ask for their prayers, but do not invite them into your life.

"Must God Heal?"

For Christians as well as nonbelievers, suffering a serious illness or watching a loved one suffer the same is extremely stressful. But the anguish is only increased when we have bought into one or more of these distortions of what Scripture actually promises. If we accept some variation of this theme that God *must always* heal, and then He doesn't, where are we? Do we deny our faith in Him?

Sometimes the frustration and desperation of what we perceive as unanswered prayer can drive us to measures that are very costly and, in some cases, unquestionably wrong. We'll look at some of these in Chapter 10.

— 10 —

The Cost of Desperation

A IDS is at present an incurable disease; the medical establishment has said it can't be cured. But people who are dying of AIDS are desperate to find something that will work. Consequently, there is a thriving underground of "treatment centers" for AIDS. All types of medications, chemicals, and machines are being used at these treatment centers, and they are all bogus. The chances of success with these clinics are about the same as your chances of winning the lottery—for all practical purposes, nonexistent.

Whenever medicine says something is hopeless and no more can be done, people become desperate. They look for something else that will give them health, some form of treatment that may offer at least a remote chance of a cure. They will go anywhere, do anything, and spend any amount.

But we will pay dearly for behavior borne of desperation. The cost may be in dollars, in time, or in comfort. The cost may be any hope of regaining health. The cost may be our witness for Jesus Christ. Sometimes, the cost may be eternal life.

Desperation May Cost You Money

One of the leading cancer researchers in our country became so frustrated with the bureaucracy of obtaining research grants for cancer that he began his own privately funded, for-profit cancer "research" institute. In most cancer research projects, the patient taking the research drug receives all treatments for free. At this "research" institute, the patient pays for everything and pays dearly.

Patients here are given the finest of medical and nursing treatment, the most medically advanced treatments available, no matter how extensive or how "far gone" the disease process is. Some treatments at least offer a glimmer of hope, though they may be totally experimental. These treatments routinely start at about thirty thousand dollars and go up from there, but there is almost a waiting list to get in this institution. Insurance doesn't pay for it; this is out-of-pocket cash in advance.

Desperation May Cost You Time

Desperation can also cost you time. Treatment means running to doctors and medical centers and treatment centers, and all that takes time.

Claire's Decision

Claire was in her late sixties when she came to see me, complaining of leg pain. Her symptoms were vague and nondescript, but troubling enough to bring her to a physician. On examination I could feel a mass in her thigh. The x-rays were negative, but the mass was definitely there and her symptoms and complaints were those of someone with a tumor.

We admitted her to the hospital and performed a biopsy. It came back revealing a highly malignant myosarcoma. She had only had the symptoms a few weeks, but this tumor was growing rapidly. It was highly malignant and, at that time, there were no treatments offering any reasonable hope for success. I called her only son, an executive in a large national Christian organization, and told him the prognosis, which was extremely grim. I felt that she had only six to nine months to live. No treatment or surgery would be successful, and any vigorous chemotherapy would only make her sick and miserable, without prolonging her life or offering any reasonable hope for cure.

Regrets

If it had been my mother, I would simply have taken her home, kept her comfortable, let her enjoy her grandchildren, and prayed for healing, because medical science had nothing realistic to offer. Instead, Claire's family took her to a major medical center where she underwent a radical operation, aggressive radiation therapy, and chemotherapy. She was miserable, sick, and suffering for five and a half months, and then she died. She had only a few good days at the beginning of that treatment.

Several years later I ran into her son. At that point he felt free to say that I had been right all along. The family regretted the loss of time they had had with their mother, but they were desperate for a cure. They had been unwilling to follow the course I had suggested.

This story also illustrates how desperation can cost a person comfort. Most radical chemotherapy and radiation routines have side affects and can make you sick and miserable. Claire's final days would probably have been much better had her family followed my advice.

Desperation May Cost You Witness

Desperation can cost us even more than time and comfort and quality of life. Living near Wheaton has given me the opportunity to treat many professing Christians. Sadly, it seems that some of the most vocal "witnesses" act in the most decidedly unChristian ways when they become desperate because of serious illness or injury. The way they behave seems to deny the very faith that they proclaim and profess. Their behavior when they are sick and desperate denies that God has the ability to heal and that God is in control and knows they are suffering.

They seek out other unproven, nonmedical treatment. They seek out illegitimate healers, false prophets, healers outside of their church, every alternative they can because they "don't want to take any chances." They behave just like the rest of pagan America. For these people, the cost of desperation becomes their visible witness for Jesus Christ.

You can profess and preach all you will, but if, when you are sick, you desperately go grabbing for any treatment you can get, rushing around in a way that denies a faith in the Almighty God who knows you, loves you, and is watching out for what is best for you, then your works will effectively destroy your witness.

Desperation May Cost You Your Life

Bobby was twenty-two when I saw him. He came in complaining of knee pains for three months. The pain was constant and waking him at night and unrelated to any activity that he did. His examination proved normal, except for some slight tenderness above his knee.

X-rays of the knee helped to reveal what appeared to be a very ominous bone tumor, probably an osteosarcoma. I told Bobby that there appeared to be something serious in the knee and brought him into the hospital for a few confirmatory tests. The tests demonstrated that there was no spread of any tumor beyond the knee, so I referred him to a medical center that specialized in the treatment of malignant bone tumors.

The treatment of these tumors in the past decade has been nothing short of spectacular. Whereas it used to be a ninety-nine percent failure rate, it is now in the seventy to eighty percent success rate in treating or curing these tumors with aggressive surgery, chemotherapy, and at times, radiation. Sometimes multiple surgeries are necessary, but they are no longer a hopeless kiss of death.

I told Bobby that I thought the had a malignant bone tumor. We did not biopsy it because at times the biopsy can affect treatment, and the treating institution is the best institution to do the biopsy. I recommended referrals for a specialist in bone tumors in Chicago and told him we could arrange treatment at the Mayo clinic or any other reputable major medical center that he would want to be transferred to.

Bobby thanked me for my concern and recommendations. He didn't question my diagnosis, but told me that his mother wasn't going to let him be treated by doctors any longer. She believed in Laitrile and knew that Laitrile would cure him. She would not permit him to have any surgery or any further medical treatment by anyone. She believed in a "cancer conspiracy" and thought doctors were withholding cures so that they could do "disfiguring surgery" and prolong treatment.

The Only Chance Rejected

I had a very frank discussion with Bobby at this point. I told him that if he did not follow my advice, the chances were he would die in less than six months. I was certain he had a highly malignant bone tumor. I certainly could not promise a successful outcome, but I felt that his only chance was to follow my advice and see a bone tumor specialist. Furthermore, I said I could get the number for him for underground Laitrile. I would not try to stop him from getting Laitrile treatments in addition to any legitimate medical and surgical treatments

At that point it was thought that Laitrile was totally harmless, and we would simply monitor him for any side effects. He thanked me for my concern, but said he doubted his mother would accept that. I offered to meet with him and his mother.

My assistant, two nurses, and a social worker attended this meeting as witnesses. We had a long, frank discussion in which I outlined the medical diagnosis and prognosis. Without treatment, I told them, I thought Bobby would be dead within six months, a year at the most. I also said that I would be glad to try and cooperate with them if they wanted Laitrile treatment in addition to the medical or surgical treatments. I also recommended referral to a major medical institution.

His mother said virtually nothing during the meeting; she just sat there like a sphinx. Several times the nurses and I asked her if she understood all I was saying, and she clearly did. That afternoon Bobby, who at twenty-two was a legal adult, signed out against medical advice. Bobby's mother never let him see me again.

She took him to Mexico to a major Laitrile clinic. They told him that he had an osteosarcoma and should go back and let Dr. Dominguez do the surgery—then they would give him the Laitrile. Since they would not treat him, Bobby's mother brought him back to the United States, where she sought out an underground Mexican nurse who treated him with a special diet, coffee ground enemas, and other noxious treatments.

The End

Five months later I was sitting in the emergency room, waiting for a patient to return from x-ray, when the ambulance crew wheeled in an obviously dying skeleton of a man. He looked worse than any victim of the Holocaust. It was Bobby, but I didn't even recognize him. He was literally breathing his last.

They called his mother and told her that if she wanted to see him alive, she had best rush to the hospital. She demanded to speak to the doctor or nurse and told them whatever they did, not to give Bobby any other food than was on his special diet. After she went to the store, she would be in. My friend told her specifically that Bobby was dying and would not be taking any nourishment of any sort through the mouth. He was already in a coma. Forty-five minutes later, the withered, emaciated skeleton of Bobby died. His mother showed up an hour later with groceries for his special diet.

Perhaps Bobby wouldn't have been cured by standard medical treatment and surgical treatment; who can say? But he would have lived longer than the five months that he did, and he would not have had to suffer the misery of repeated daily coffee ground enemas and an unpalatable medical diet. And Bobby might very well have been cured. Bobby blew it. It cost him his life!

Whom Do You Believe?

Bobby's mother was an avid reader of the tabloids,

those sleazy magazines that for years have bandied headlines about the "cancer conspiracy." According to these magazines, cancer physicians and surgeons, cancer hospitals and institutes, and cancer radiation therapists are all profiting from the treatment of cancer and would all be out of business if cancer were cured. Because of this fear of the cures for cancer which "are already available," these doctors are supposedly supressing word of these cures. Doctors could cure cancer, but they don't, because they can make more money doing surgery and prolonging the suffering.

Of course there is no cancer conspiracy. As soon as a cure for any type of cancer is known, it is widely published and used by legitimate physicians everywhere.

Satan's Offer

Just as Satan tempted Christ and offered Him all the kingdoms of the earth and all the wealth of the earth, Satan makes offers to us, telling us that false prophets and false healers have the ability to heal us. But the Bible asks, "What shall it profit a man if he gain the whole world and lose his soul?" (Mark 8:36) Believers who seek out false prophets or healers may be healed, but it is a Faustian pact that they are making.

Some say if you're desperate, no price is too high for even the slightest hope of a cure. And if you buy the philosophy and religion of American paganism, that's true. If you're only "looking out for number one," if you "only go around once," if you "have to grab every moment," then that's true. But for the believer, who doesn't buy into American paganism, the cost of desperation is too high.

11

Healing That
Doesn't Glorify God

I was flying home from the Olympic training center at Colorado, having participated in a coaches' clinic there. I was reading a book by J. I. Packer. A coach asked me what I was doing. When I said I was reading a book about the Holy Spirit in preparation for my Sunday school class on faith healing, I instantly had the attention of everyone in the surrounding seats. Faith healing is a topic everyone wants to know about.

A coach from Oregon, who was sitting next to me, said his next door neighbor had flown to the Philippines to see a psychic surgeon. The man had been diagnosed and treated for cancer and in desperation flew to the Philippines. He related that his neighbor had undergone successful psychic surgery and the big tumor had been removed from him. Ten weeks later, the man died of the cancer.

Psychic surgery is just one type of healing that doesn't glorify God. In this chapter we will see several types of these healers and will examine the criteria the scripture gives for judging whether a faith healer is legitimately from God.

Psychic Surgeons

Psychic surgeons are one type of false prophet abounding in our world today. They appear to remove organs, tumors, and blood clots from people, but in truth they are fakers.

Tony was a world famous, world class tennis player. He developed tendonitis in his elbow which affected his ability to play, and he began to lose matches. He consulted orthopedic surgeons in many countries who had many treatments including cortisone injections. His elbow continued to get worse.

He finally chose a world famous orthopedic surgeon who performed surgery on his elbow. He was no better after the surgery. A year and a half later he was still disabled with elbow pain and unable to play competitive tennis. In desperation, he flew to the Philippines to see a famous psychic surgeon. Some of his entourage went with him. Tony was too squeamish to watch what the psychic surgeon did. He said that all that he felt was a hot flash in his elbow and a tingling, and the pain went away. He was totally relieved. He returned to world class competitive level for two and a half more years and enjoyed success.

His friends who were with him said that it appeared that the psychic surgeon had opened up his elbow, and removed all the clotted blood and damaged tissue, and then closed it back up. This was all done in a matter of seconds, just with his hand—no scalpel, no nothing.

Out and Out Fakers

The psychic surgeons of the Philippines are world famous. Investigative journalists have proven that psychic surgeons are masters of sleight of hand. The blood clots they remove are clotted goat or sheep blood. At times they will open up abdomens and take out organs; and these organs are chicken or goat or sheep organs which are reported to be tumors. When the psychic surgeons lift out a bloody mass of tissue, most untrained people are incapable of looking closely at what happens. The investigative journalists, by their own "sleight of hand," obtained some of this tissue and blood to test it scientifically. It always proved to be animal blood of some sort, not human.

Psychic surgeons are out-and-out fakers, profiteers. They are false prophets, though it is important to note that some may be miraculously cured by their efforts. Remember that Satan is also in the miracle business. He is the great deceiver. He is not as powerful as God, but he is the prince of the earth. Our tendency even as Christians to deny Satan's existence and his power is simply another example of how we have succumbed to the subtle influences of American paganism.

The Witch Doctor

George was the chronic VA patient. He was constantly trying to be admitted to the Seattle VA hospital because he was convinced he had a brain tumor and was dying. Furthermore, whenever George was in the hospital, his benefits were increased. He made more money in the hospital than he did out.

George was a master of deception, and knew all the right symptoms to claim. Any gullible neurosurgical resident who was not familiar with his background, would certainly admit him into the hospital. Once in the hospital, it would take nearly an act of Congress to get him out.

This scenario had been repeated over and over and over again. George realized when the residents would change rotation. He had a chance of catching a new resident on call once every six to twelve months, and then he could con his way into the hospital.

Once again George had caught a new resident, stated his symptoms, and been admitted for work up for a brain tumor. The work up was being speeded up to hustle George out of the hospital, when one morning George was found dead in his bed. The residents were horrified. An autopsy was ordered and was completely negative. There was no medical explanation for George's death. There was no brain tumor. There was no brain cancer. George should have been alive!

It turned out that in the room next to George there was a man, a devout Roman Catholic, dying of brain cancer. The priest was summoned in the middle of the night to give last rites to this man. In typical VA fashion, the priest was told "third door on your right." The poor bleary-eyed priest, walking down the corridor at two-thirty in the morning, miscounted doors. He walked into George's room and administered the last rites to George. That is the last time anyone saw George alive.

The only explanation that could be given for George's death was that being awakened in the middle of the night and given the last rites literally scared George to death! Convinced that he was dying, the fear and apprehension killed him.

The Power of Suggestion

Almost every missionary returning from a culture that has witch doctors has a similar story. The witch doctor would put a curse on a perfectly normal, healthy person. That person will tell the missionary that he has been cursed and is going to die in a certain number of days or weeks and, sure enough, right on schedule the person becomes sick. The missionary doctors can't diagnose him or treat him, and the person dies on schedule.

Witch doctors have enormous power and control over their people. Much of this control, if not all of it, is through the people's fear and belief in the witch doctors' power. But witch doctors also have some potent agents at their disposal. Smoke is a prominent part of many pagan rituals, and the material being smoked is not usually tobacco—it's marijuana. What better way to have peace among warriors than to calm them down by smoking a potent tranquilizer or other strong drugs and hallucinogens! Witch doctors have used "strong medicine" in every culture.

"Good" witch doctors or good parapsychologists also know their plants well enough to recognize those which had medicinal benefits. These witch doctors are able to treat certain ailments and infections by applying poultices or administering certain herbs and drugs with some success.

Pact With the Devil

But witch doctors are the modern day, third world equivalent of a Dr. Faustus. They have made their pact with the devil. They have success over magic and are able to control people's minds and leave them distraught. Most of us in our culture don't put much faith in witch doctors; we don't appreciate the power they have over their people's minds, the immense fear and awe they are held in, and the enormous power Satan gives them.

In an "intellectual" and "enlightened" society, witch

doctors usually do not wield a great deal of control. It is supposed to take ignorance and superstition to give them their power. But with the rise of Satanism and devil worship in our country, one has to wonder about these smug assumptions. Do not be fooled. Satan is alive and well and flourishing in the world. He is just more overt in "less Christian" countries.

While witch doctors can treat some physical ills, their main concern is the spiritual battle. We may be more sophisticated and more intellectual, but the witch doctors have known that all along that the real war is over men's spirits and their minds.

False Prophets "In the Name of Jesus"

Stories of psychic healers and witch doctors may be interesting, but most of us don't feel particularly threatened by them. "Isn't is good that we're not that gullible," we reassure ourselves. "How pathetic to be part of such an unenlightened culture."

But for the evangelical Christian in the United States, there is another false prophet, a wolf in sheep's clothing, ready to take advantage of us when we're most vulnerable. It is the person who claims to speak for God, but who is doing it for some reason other than the love of God.

Elmer Gantry

Elmer Gantry is the story of an itinerant evangelist and "faith healer" who traveled around the country holding tent meetings and healing services—all for profit. Elmer Gantry was a faker, and there are many like him around.

How do today's Gantrys operate? There are many

ways to fake healing. One of the easiest is to have employees stir up the crowd by pretending they have been healed miraculously, and then rely on emotion and mass hysteria to evoke other examples of healing from innocent attenders.

A more subtle way is to have a staff member interview sick people as they limp into the service, hoping to be healed. In this way they gain valuable information: name, malady, treatment, doctors' names, etc. Then, in the emotion of the service, the fake healer (through the aid of a hidden walkie talkie or ear plug) is able to name the sick person's name, their malady, what treatments they had, even the name of their doctor. In all honesty they can ask the sick person, "Have I ever met you? Have you ever told me these things?" The answer, of course, is no. At this point they may have forgotten the "innocent" incoming interview.

Another trick is having attendants offer wheelchairs to frail or elderly people as they come in, so they can sit down in front. Later the healer lays hands on them and tells them to get up. Of course they can—they were simply wheeled to the front "for a better view." But the rest of this congregation thinks these people were wheelchair bound.

Who Is Legitimate?

So how can we judge which faith healers are legitimate and which are frauds? Scripture has given us two clear criteria.

First, is a fee or gift required to see the healer? If so, then the healer is a false prophet, a faker. The strongest condemnations in the Bible were those who healed by invoking the name of Jesus for a profit. Simon the sor-

cerer was condemned strongly by Peter for wanting the
gift for profit. In Acts 19:13, seven sons of a Jewish
priest, Sceva, were trying to drive out evil spirits in the
name of Jesus for profit. They were attacked, physically
beaten, and forced to run through the streets naked.

By contrast, anyone with a true gift of healing gives of
it freely.

The second test to use for false prophets is the message they preach. Is Jesus Christ named as the son of
God? Many people will invoke the name of Jesus, but
that alone is not enough. It is the entire message that
has to be judged. Is Christ, as God, lifted up? Is He the
main reason for the services?

Remember that the Elmer Gantrys may produce miraculous results. Matthew 7:15-23 clearly documents
that false prophets can perform miracles. But "this is
how you can recognize the Spirit of God: Every spirit
that acknowledges that Jesus Christ has come in the
flesh is from God. But every spirit that does not acknowledge Jesus is not from God." (I John 4:1). The lit-
mus test is not the illnesses healed, but whether Jesus
Christ is acknowledged as the Son of God.

12

Bringing Healing
to Each Other

How, you may wonder, could sincere, devout Christians ever be deceived into pursuing healing through the bizarre and evil counterfeits described in the last chapter? Perhaps one reason is that we as a church have failed to do our part in bringing healing to each other. Scripture exhorts us repeatedly to bear each other's burdens. Many of us have a latent "gift of healing" that is exercised by caring, talking, and supporting those who are ill.

In many inner city areas of America, there are small charismatic storefront churches, one to a block or sometimes more, depending on the density of the population. The congregations in these churches average thirty to forty people. Typically, if it gets larger than that, a new church is formed. When one of their members is ill or injured, these vibrant, alive churches respond immediately with practical help for the injured person. They visit at the hospital. They visit at home. They bring over food. They help with childcare. They function as a complete body of Christ in which each member has a different task, and no member tries to go it alone.

In our large churches we have lost that. It is possible for someone to be in the hospital two weeks, and no one will know about it. It is possible for someone to be out of church a month and not be missed.

Mobilize the Forces

Here are some practical ways we as Christians can bring healing to each other. First, mobilize the forces. Don't keep an illness a secret—it's not gossiping to let friends and church members know that someone is ill! Let them know who is sick and what is happening. You need to rally their support and assistance.

I'm still amazed at the number of people who think that I, as a physician attending the hospital, know the name and room number of every patient admitted the night before. I've made rounds on the same floor where someone from my church was hospitalized, and didn't know it until their name jumped out at me from a chart.

Be practical. Cards and flowers are great, but if the mother of small children is sick, it is obvious the family will need help with childcare. If the parents are having to commute into a medical center for treatment, meals may be necessary. Someone may need to help clean the house or mow the grass. If the ailing person is a senior citizen, a ride to the doctor's office may be what's needed. The point is to help physically in any way that you can.

Call on the Sick Person

Call on the sick person. While the telephone is a wonderful invention, it can also be a cop out. Many people are reluctant to visit people in the hospital. While this is a common fear, it is unrealistic. People in the hospital are generally alone and want visitors. Ten to fifteen minutes is the most time that you need to spend; any longer may be too tiring for the patient.

You don't need to be afraid you're going to catch something. If the person has something contagious, there are usually big warning signs plastered all over the doors or windows or signs saying stop at the nurse's station before you visit. But even then, it is usually safe to visit after you stop and get instructions. They may require that you wear a gown and gloves or a gown and mask.

Actually, most of the time, people have to wear gowns and masks to prevent the patient from catching the bugs that you have, rather than the other way around. It's because their resistance is down, and you may contaminate them.

Be Willing to Listen

Many people are afraid to visit the sick because they won't know what to say. This is especially true if it's a serious illness. So you will no longer have that excuse, I am going to tell you right now the answer to that feeling. It is this: no one knows what to say.

Be truthful. Tell them you don't know what to say. You can say you are sorry they are sick, or you understand they are suffering a great loss. You realize they must be in pain and you feel bad for them.

Anyone can express sympathy for a person who is hurting. But if you've ever experienced the same illness or a similar injury or loss, then you really have something to share. Years ago, I tried to console a mother who had suddenly lost her son in an accident. I said something like, "I know the suffering you're going through."

"How can you know?" she retorted angrily. "Have you ever lost a son?"

No, I hadn't. I felt chastened and chagrined. I began then to realize how important empathy is. If you have suffered a similar loss and can be empathetic, God can use that special gift to bring healing to others.

Joe Bayly and his wife, Mary Lou, suffered the loss of not one, not two, but three sons over a period of time, all from different causes. Out of this caldron of grief and loss, Joe wrote several books and he became an "expert" on the Christian perspective on grief and dying. He and Mary Lou developed that superior kind of sympathy that we've talked about—empathy.

No one could say they had not suffered loss or felt pain. They had been there, so they understood. They did not turn their grief and loss into anger, but to the Lord's will.

When my nephew Ace died, I asked the Baylys to talk with Marge and Ray, Ace's parents. I had said all I could say to my sister and her husband; I could sympathize with them, but I could not empathize.

Joe and Mary Lou met with Marge and Ray several times. Both Marge and Ray grew spiritually from these meetings; they both relate that Joe and Mary Lou were the single most important people in helping them deal with their grief.

Be Willing to Serve

But even if you haven't suffered, you can be a listener. Few of us have the experience of the Baylys, but all of us can exercise the gift of healing by giving the suffering person an opportunity to be heard. You'd be surprised how many people want to talk, and how few want to listen.

I'd been in practice for a few years and was making hospital rounds one day when I was paged. It was Judy, my wife. Seven months pregnant, she called me from home to say she was dizzy and uncoordinated and couldn't even crawl to the bathroom, because she would fall over to one side.

Too uncoordinated and dizzy to crawl! I dashed home and brought her into the hospital, where it was soon clear that she had encephalitis. We had four little ones at home at the time.

In the hospital, Judy's condition deteriorated daily. Medicine had done all that it could, and it did not appear that Judy was going to survive. Her headaches became so severe that for three days straight she begged me to kill her. (She denies this, but that is because she, fortunately, does not remember any of those three days.)

Throughout this time people would come up and ask me how my wife was doing. The only honest statement was that she was doing worse, thank you for asking. But after two days of answering this way, it became painful for me to be honest because of the obvious discomfort it caused the people who asked. So for twelve days in a row, I lied. I would say, "Thank you, she's doing better." They didn't really want to know.

We're all like that. None of us wants to hear bad news; we'd rather flee from it. But that's not the Christian way; that's not the healing way. What we need to do is to honestly express, "I'm sorry to hear that. I'm hurting for you. Is there anything I can do to help?" And then *listen*—don't cut them off.

Listening can be costly. You may discover problems or find out about tangible needs that must be met—and you may have to help meet them. But doesn't being a follower of Christ involve some cost?

There is also a small risk, but it should be mentioned, that you might find yourself being manipulated by the patient. The sufferer may become overly dependent on you. While it's important for us to love and be helpful and listen and do things to help, we cannot do everything for people. Just as children can't be carried all the time or they won't learn to walk, so at times some people who are recovering from illnesses must be forced to fend for themselves in order to complete their healing.

If you find yourself being caught in a web of doing too much for someone, talk it over with a friend and see what they think. If they think you are being used or manipulated, you may have to take steps to resolve the problem. But frankly, the problem is hardly ever that of doing too much—it is usually the reverse, that we don't do enough.

Be Willing to Touch

One of the best things to come out of Hollywood was the hug or a kiss on the cheek as a greeting. Hugging and touching and kissing are normal, natural ways that loved ones greet each other.

In our churches today, we see very little touching and much less hugging and kissing. But it's Biblical to "greet one another with a kiss of love" (I Peter 5:14). It is ironic that there is so little show of physical affection amongst brothers and sisters in Christ in this day and age of "sexual liberation."

Nevertheless, there is something very special about touching and holding hands when you are visiting with someone who is ill. If you feel moved to do it, hug them. Especially when you're hurting, there's nothing like a hug. It's interesting to note how many times Christ touched a person He was healing. Touching is potent medicine.

If you're not convinced, think about one of the real giant strides in medicine the last decade, the care and nurturing of preemies in pediatric neonatology. Babies like those for whom there was no hope when I was in training are now routinely nurtured and brought to full and complete lives. Yet with all medical advances, all the monitors and incubators and intravenous solutions and respirators for treating these minute human beings, there is one essential tool that you'll see in every preemie nursery—the rocking chair.

When I was in medical school, these little babies were left in their isolettes, not touched by human hands. Although they received some of the same life-giving treatments preemies now receive, they all died. The difference now is that the nursery nurses are encouraged to pick up the babies, handle them, fondle them, and rock them. The parents are encouraged to come in and hold their babies and rock them. It's the human touch that's the critical tool to healing.

Be Willing to Pray

Before you end your hospital visits, ask the patients if they want you to pray with them. If they say yes, hold their hands or put your arm around them and pray. Pray for relief from pain and suffering. Pray for strength to endure. Pray for healing. Pray that God will reach through their suffering and speak with them and show them His will for them.

Don't be judgmental and pray for forgiveness of their sins that caused them to be ill. Don't pray that they will no longer be punished. Don't pray that they will have enough faith to be healed. We are to bear one another's burdens, not be a burden or add to their stress. Don't question their faith or tell them they need to get right with God and everything is going to be okay. They may be more "right with God" than you.

If they don't want you to pray with them now, though I think this is highly unlikely, then you need to honor their request. They are depriving themselves of an enormous source of healing and power, because Christ has promised He will be present where two or more of us are gathered together and praying in His name.

Tell them when you are leaving that you are going to pray for them—and then do it.

"See How They Love One Another!"

We've been assuming that the person whom you are visiting is a Christian. Suggestions about practical health, talking and listening, touching and hugging, apply as well to the non-believer—especially to your neighbor, co-worker, or someone else you know reasonably well. We need to demonstrate Christ's love to others whether or not they are fellow believers.

If you are visiting an unbeliever, you can still be a practical help. You can talk and be a good listener and touch or hug them. When you're done with the visit, tell them you are going to pray for them. I believe that is always appropriate. I have never yet met anyone, even an atheist, who is offended or turned off by an offer of prayer when they are hurting, sick, or injured. Most people, regardless of their faith or stated belief, are thankful for that kind of offer.

Having made that offer, don't dash out the door. Give

them the chance to ask you to pray for them now. If that happens, acknowledge in your prayer that God is hearing your prayers and that He is a God who loves this person, cares for him or her, and knows of this suffering. Pray for relief from pain, pray for healing, and pray for any other items of concern that came up in your conversation earlier. This will communicate that no concern is too small for God.

Again, don't be judgmental. Don't preach at them in prayer. Pray for their concerns and requests. Remember, it is the Holy Spirit who convicts of sin, and not us. We are called only to demonstrate Christ's love.

All people who are sick and suffering like to be told that they haven't been forgotten and that someone cares about them. Through helping out, through visiting, listening, touching, and praying, we tangibly demonstrate that we do care for each other. May our world say of the Church, "See, how they love one another!"

13

Glorifying God

Let me tell you the story of Louise, a Christian who was sick "the right way." Louise is a lovely, devout Christian woman. Several years ago she noted a change in her bowel habit. After several months of knowing something wrong, and six weeks of having blood in her stool, she finally mentioned it to me. I instantly thought of colon cancer and strongly recommended that she see a "real doctor" for a consultation and surgery.

Louise and her church were praying, first of all that the symptoms would go away, and second that the test would turn out negative. A barium enema was ordered and confirmed the presence of a large "mass" at the upper end of the colon. It was so large that it was going to block colon function so, rather than biopsying it first, the doctor felt it was most expeditious to proceed with surgery, even in the unlikely event that the mass would turn out to be benign.

To my relief, Louise consented to the surgery. I had seen Christians refuse surgery under these circumstances, or at least delay the decision longer than they should. But she and her church prayed that the surgery would go well and that the mass would be benign. Louise was convinced that it could not be cancerous.

The tumor was malignant, but the surgery went well. The surgeon was convinced he "got it all," and he was sure that the operation was successful and no further treatment, either radiation or chemotherapy, would be necessary.

But when the pathology report came back, the tumor was revealed to be an unusual type of colon cancer, much more malignant than typical. It was already invading the wall of the colon, and there was a high likelihood that it would spread if radiation treatment were not performed.

This was a shock to all concerned. Louise, her surgeon, and I attended the conference between the cancer specialist, the oncologist, the pathologist, and the radiation therapist, and it was clear that this was the best recommendation. Louise underwent a course of radiation treatments that progressed without a hitch.

During the initial illness, Louise wasn't worried at all, because she "knew" she didn't have cancer. But once the diagnosis was firmly established, she began to worry a bit. She admitted that, for several years following the radiation treatment, she felt apprehension each time she went in for a check-up. But throughout the illness, Louise's faith never wavered.

From the moment she first talked to me, I knew Louise had cancer. Her symptoms were textbook. She has been totally healed and is now free of cancer—I'm convinced of that. But of more importance to me is the fact that Louise's response to her illness was never at odds with her profession of faith. I had seen it happen so often the other way that I was especially relieved when this particular saint didn't let me down, for Louise is my mother.

The Positive, Christian Approach

As Louise's story demonstrates, even a potentially fatal illness doesn't have to drag you down and depress you. There are many positive things you can do if you become sick or disabled. How you react to this time of stress has a lot to do with how quickly you will recover.

The following list is not "ten easy steps to healing," or anything like it. Rather, it's a reiterating of some important truths we've discussed throughout this book, summarized in brief paragraphs.

1. Remember that God is in control.

We learn from Christ's miracles that God has the ability to heal; no case is "hopeless." There is a God who loves you and cares for you and wants you to be healthy.

This fact alone is very comforting. Nonbelievers do not have access to this positive assurance that there is a God who is in control and who loves and cares for them.

2. Pray about your illness.

Tell God you're sick and ask to be healed. Philippians 4:6 says, "Do not be anxious about anything, but in everything, by prayer and petition, with thanksgiving, present your requests to God." God knows we're sick, but we are still commanded to come before Him and ask for healing. Remember there is an enormous power in prayer and you need to really know that God can heal you and then pray for it. Once you do that, you mobilize your immune system and your own recuperative powers. This is an essential part of getting better.

3. Get others to help pray.

Be open and frank with your friends at church. We are commanded to pray for each others' burdens. The Bible says where two or three are gathered together, God will be present. There is more power where two or three Christians are present than when one person prays alone. You're not tapping into the true power line if you don't share your needs with your Christian brothers and sisters.

Remember also James 5:14. Don't hesitate to call the elders or deacons and ask them to pray over you and lay their hands on you.

4. Don't forget the mud, spit, and fingers of medical science.

If, in your illness today, you could come before a physical, living Christ and ask him to heal you, wouldn't you follow his instructions? If he spit in the dirt and smeared mud on your face and told you to walk through town and wash it off in the public fountain in the town square, wouldn't you do it? Or would you run to the nearest shower instead?

Western medicine has much to offer and can do many miraculous things. Failing to make use of it is like rejecting Christ's instructions; if the blind beggar had refused Christ's mud and spit, he would probably not have been healed.

5. Learn some lessons.

It is now time to meditate and contemplate and pray that God will open your eyes to the lessons to be learned from this illness. Is He beating you over the head with a two-by-four to get your attention? Do you need to slow down or to pay less attention to the things of this earth and more attention to spiritual things? Many a spiritual wakening and change of life direction has occurred during illness.

Make the most of your illness or disability. Whatever

you do, listen for the still small voice of God. He is in control. He is going to make the best use of your illness, even if you don't want to be sick. God knows you're sick; He knows you're hurting. He may want you to be sick for a while.

6. Remember that nonbelievers may be watching you.

Maybe you are ill simply to give you the opportunity to be a witness for them. God does have a plan, and your illness somehow fits into that plan whether or not you ever know the explanation. God will make the most of your illness for His kingdom and for your ultimate benefit.

7. Don't doubt your faith because you are sick.

Remember, it may be *because* of your faith that you are sick. It may not become obvious until years from now, or it may never become obvious to you, but God will use this to further His kingdom.

Furthermore, remember that you will not be tested above that which you are able (I Corinthians 10:13). You have the faith to see this through.

8. Don't think you are being punished.

It is very rare, as we've pointed out, for Christians to be punished with illness. And in all instances where they were punished, they were warned loudly and forcefully about their sin and the impending punishment, and they knew the warning was correct. So don't let "friends" or acquaintances drag you down by telling you you're being punished.

9. Don't be impatient.

We are creatures of the clock, a goal-oriented and time-conscious people. We are frustrated with waiting, and we see delay as failure. Remember, time consciousness is a cultural thing that we've learned; it's part of our "McDonald's mentality." Any time you put time demands on God, you are going to be frustrated. His "clock" is entirely different from ours. God does not heal the way they serve food at McDonald's, but God does answer prayer.

10. Don't demand that God remove the thorn.

Remember that Paul prayed three times that God would remove the thorn in his flesh, but he was told that the thorn was there for his own good. "My grace is sufficient for you," God told him.

You don't *need* it removed. God can do his work better in an imperfect physical specimen; the thorn in the flesh may be there for your own good and for the good of the Kingdom.

Ace's Homegoing

I have seen a lot of people die. Death and dying go with the territory of being a physician. There is, however, one death I still cannot relate without a crack in my voice or breaking down in tears.

Ace was the only child of my sister and brother-in-law's marriage. He was a beautiful child, beautiful in countenance and beautiful in spirit. At one and a half, Ace was dying.

The church prayed for him. The elders of the church anointed him with oil. But after two major cancer operations, chemotherapy, and radiation therapy, medical science had nothing more to offer. At Children's Memorial Hospital, they frantically treated him anyhow. The treatments were unpleasant. Ace was hooked up to tubes and IV's.

His mother had the courage and compassion to ask why; was there any hope? Told that there was none, she said, "I am taking him home."

The nurses related later that they'd expected Ace to die within twenty-four hours. But the family gathered. Ace was held, non-stop, for two and a half weeks. He took virtually no sustenance and was continually in pain. Occasionally he responded to his mother. There has never been a more graphic demonstration of the power of touch and hugging and caring and love.

At the end of that two and a half week period, it became clear that death was imminent. Ace had been barely breathing for almost twenty-four hours and was not responding at all. We gathered around him in my sister's bedroom, where she was holding this frail, wasted child.

He hadn't spoken in over a week, and for that matter hadn't done much more than moan and roll his eyes. For twenty-four hours he had not responded to anything. His breathing was very erratic. Suddenly Ace sat up in his mother's arms, pointed directly upwards to a corner of the room, and said in a clear, loud voice, "See, Mommy, see?" Over and over again he said it.

His mother said, "What, Ace?" The windows were closed in the room, but we all felt a definite cool breeze and a presence. There was an electricity, a charge in the room that was palpable.

"See, Mommy, see?" Ace said, with a smile on his face. And he died.

None of the ten adults in that room had any question that at least an angel had come to take Ace home. For Ace, death was wonderful. His trials and sufferings were over. He was with his grandfather and his uncle.

The Victory

I am not a mystic, but that was a mystical experience. It was life changing and faith confirming—one of the most beautiful things that I have ever experienced. Nevertheless, it did not ease the pain of having to carry the lifeless body of my nephew out of the house to the undertaker. It did not ease the pain that my sister and brother-in-law felt, nor did it ease their loss.

Death is horrible—for those left behind. But if we truly believe what the Bible says, it is not horrible for those who have died. As the apostle Paul says, "For to me, to live is Christ. And to die, is to gain" (Philippians 1:21).

It is Paul again who reminds us that we don't see the big picture. We are looking through fogged glass, "through a glass darkly." If we could see the whole picture, the truly grand design of not only our lives, but the interworking and interrelationships of ourselves to others and God's working in history, then we would understand, and it would all make sense. For now, we must believe with the psalmist that "precious in the sight of the Lord is the death of His saints" (Psalms 116:15).

The Book of Common Prayer contains a prayer "that we may end our lives in faith and hope, without suffering and without reproach." This is the way that Christians should face death, for death for believers is transition to new life—*whole* life—eternal life.

"I heard a voice from heaven say, 'Write: blessed are the dead who die in the Lord from now on.' 'Yes,' sayeth the spirit, 'They will rest from their labor, for their deeds follow them'" (Revelation 14:13).

There is a gracious way to die. There is a glorious way to die. There is a Christian way to die.

Yes, God wants His children to be healthy. We are to glorify Him in our health, serve Him in our health, and worship Him in our health. It is one of the ways that He blesses us. But it is not the only way. We can also glory in our suffering, knowing that God's strength is made perfect in our weakness. God will use our sufferings to bring us closer to Him.

One final thought from Paul, a verse that has colored the way I view my life: "I have learned that in whatsoever state I'm in, therewith to be content" (Philippians 4:11). God is great, and He blesses us in whatever state we're in.